To my children
Amelia, Toby and Connie
and in memory of their mother
Andrea Marguerite Cobon

Lecture Notes
Neurology

Lionel Ginsberg

BSc, MB, BS, PhD, FRCP
Consultant Neurologist, Royal Free Hospital, London;
Honorary Consultant Physician, National Hospital for
Neurology and Neurosurgery, Queen Square, London;
Clinical Sub-Dean and Welfare Tutor, Royal Free Campus,
University College London Medical School, London

Ninth Edition

WILEY-BLACKWELL

A John Wiley & Sons, Ltd., Publication

Library of Congress Cataloging-in-Publication Data

Ginsberg, Lionel.
  Lecture notes. Neurology / Lionel Ginsberg. – 9th ed.
    p. ; cm.
  Includes bibliographical references and index.
  ISBN 978-1-4051-7722-1
  1. Neurology.   I. Title.   II. Title: Neurology.
  [DNLM: 1. Nervous System Diseases. WL 140 G493L 2010]
  RC346.G56 2005
  616.8–dc22
                                        2009038758

ISBN: 9781405177221

A catalogue record for this book is available from the British Library.

Set in 8/12pt Stone Serif by Aptara® Inc., New Delhi, India
Printed and bound in Malaysia by Vivar Prinitng Sdn Bhd

1   2010

Contents

Preface to the ninth edition

The seventh edition of *Lecture Notes on Neurology* involved a complete revision of the text, an opportunity afforded by the change of author. With the eighth and ninth editions, there have been further refinements as follows:

• Selected case histories, drawn from life, are given at the end of each chapter in Part 2 of the book, so that important clinical points made in the main text can be illustrated and expanded.

• A series of sample examination questions and answers is given at the end of the volume. Desmond Kidd, Consultant Neurologist, and Thomas Solbach, Consultant Neuroradiologist, kindly provided figures to accompany some of these questions.

• Some of the figures in the main text have been replaced and a few new ones added.

• The text has been fully updated to reflect the continuing rapid advances in neurological management.

Tony Wilson and Charlie Davie, Consultant Neurologists, kindly read and commented on the case histories and examination questions, respectively. Susan Huson, Consultant Clinical Geneticist, commented on Table 18.3. Editorial staff at Wiley-Blackwell, notably Laura Murphy and Karen Moore, were patient and tolerant as always. Final thanks must again go to Sue, my wife, for her encouragement and support.

Lionel Ginsberg

Preface to the seventh edition

More than a decade has passed since the sixth edition of Dr Ivan Draper's *Lecture Notes on Neurology*. This seventh edition has been prepared with the dual aims of reflecting advances in neurology in the intervening period and changes in the undergraduate medical curriculum.

There have been dramatic developments in neurological practice in recent years, paralleling achievements in basic neuroscience research. These include new imaging techniques, which have greatly refined diagnostic accuracy and spared patients the discomfort of previous investigative approaches. Novel therapies are beginning to appear for conditions once considered untreatable. Molecular genetic research has cast new light on disease pathogenesis and should ultimately pay dividends in the treatment, as well as diagnosis, of inherited disorders.

Despite these advances, neurology remains *par excellence* a clinical discipline. Contrary to popular opinion outside the specialty, it is not a sterile and obscure diagnostic exercise. Neurological disorders are common, permeating the whole of general medicine and surgery. Their diagnosis is based on accurate history-taking and physical examination, coupled with the application of logical rules derived from knowledge of the underlying anatomy, physiology and pathology.

This volume is intended to emphasize these general principles. In line with the concept of an undergraduate 'core curriculum', it also concentrates on common diseases. The book falls naturally into two parts. The first section, 'The Neurological Approach', is concerned with history-taking and examination, where possible linked to relevant anatomy and physiology. A final chapter in this part outlines the expanding range of neurological investigations. The second section, 'Neurological Disorders', is a systematic account of the common conditions, rarities being relegated to the tables, or to a brief thumbnail sketch. There are also chapters on neurological emergencies, neurorehabilitation and the interface between neurology and other specialties. The separation of general from systematic is incomplete. For convenience, some disorders are discussed in the first part of the book and some principles appear for the first time in the second. The author also apologizes for occasions where his enthusiasm has allowed discussion of a few topics that might be considered beyond the range of a 'core curriculum'. Their inclusion may, it is hoped, be justified on grounds of continuity and interest, particularly where they reflect growing areas of neurological research and practice.

This new edition of *Lecture Notes on Neurology* should function as a portable companion during a student's neurology clinical attachment, and also senior medical clerkships. It may serve as a revision aid, and contains a grounding for early postgraduate work in general medicine.

Lionel Ginsberg

Acknowledgements

This work would not have been completed without the secretarial assistance of Barbara Parker, who uncomplainingly coped with numerous drafts and corrections. Many colleagues read selected chapters. I am grateful to Bob Bradford, Consultant Neurosurgeon, Heather Angus-Leppan, Jeremy Gibbs, John Hodges, Gareth Llewelyn, Gordon Plant, Tony Schapira, Neil Scolding, Tom Warner and Tony Wilson, Consultant Neurologists, for their comments. The responsibility for any remaining errors is, of course, my own. Several student reviewers at Blackwell Publishing also made helpful suggestions, which have been incorporated wherever possible. The editorial staff at Blackwell Publishing, particularly Mike Stein and Andrew Robinson, have been embodiments of patience and tolerance.

Most of the radiological figures were kindly provided by Alan Valentine, Consultant Neuroradiologist. Figure 10.1 was from the Department of Clinical Neurophysiology at the Royal Free Hospital. Pathological plates were prepared by Jim McLaughlin, Consultant Neuropathologist. The Department of Medical Illustration at the Royal Free Hospital helped provide most of the clinical photographs. Several other figures were prepared by Kieran Price. Finally, I thank my wife, Sue, who encouraged and supported me, and drafted most of the line drawings.

Lionel Ginsberg

Part 1

The Neurological Approach

Chapter 1

Neurological history-taking

The diagnosis and management of diseases of the nervous system have been revolutionized in recent years by new techniques of investigation and new treatments. But neurology continues to rely as much as any other branch of medicine on the fundamental clinical skills of history-taking and physical examination.

Neurological diagnosis

The neurological diagnosis is generally separable into two parts:
- Anatomical: What is the site of the lesion in the nervous system?
- Pathological: What disease process has occurred at that site?

This division is helpful as it can reduce possible confusion caused by the many available sites for neurological disorder (Table 1.1).

The history is of paramount importance in determining both the anatomical and pathological diagnoses. Indeed, many neurological patients have no abnormal signs, or simply have physical features that confirm clinical suspicions based on the history.

Sometimes, however, particularly with complex problems, the history can only yield a 'shortlist' of potential sites of the lesion(s) and final local-

Table 1.1 Potential sites of neurological disease.

Cerebral cortex
Cerebral white matter
Basal ganglia
Cerebellum
Brainstem
Cranial nerves
Spinal cord
Spinal roots
Peripheral nerves
Neuromuscular junction
Muscle

ization must await the formal examination. This is because disease at one site in the nervous system may produce symptoms mimicking a lesion at another.

History of presenting complaint

How can the history best be taken to provide the maximum diagnostic information? An important rule is first to allow the patient sufficient uninterrupted time to speak. Most patients can give a reasonable account of their symptoms within 2 or 3 minutes and time spent listening at this stage is not wasted.

The nature of the main complaint and its duration will usually have been established in this early part of the interview, along with three further essential pieces of information about the patient:

Lecture Notes: Neurology, 9th edition. By Lionel Ginsberg. Published 2010 by Blackwell Publishing.

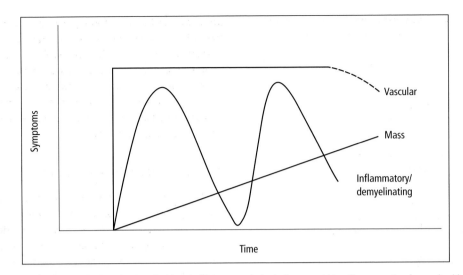

Figure 1.1 Temporal patterns associated with specific neuropathological causes. Using the example of a cerebral hemisphere lesion presenting with contralateral weakness, a rapid onset (seconds, minutes or at most hours) and static subsequent course, ultimately possibly with some improvement, suggest a vascular event (**stroke**), i.e. haemorrhage or infarction. A slowly progressive course (days, weeks or months) is more indicative of a **mass** lesion, i.e. a tumour. A relapsing and remitting pattern (with symptoms typically developing and resolving over days or weeks, then perhaps recurring with a similar time course) generally implies a **chronic inflammatory** or **demyelinating** process, of which multiple sclerosis is the prime example in the central nervous system.

- Age
  - Certain neurological disorders are associated with specific age groups.
- Occupation
  - A patient may have experienced occupational exposure to a toxin or other potential causative agent of disease.
  - Some neurological symptoms may limit the patient's ability to perform certain occupations.
- Handedness
  - To obtain information about cerebral hemisphere dominance.
  - To establish the extent to which a patient is disabled if the presenting complaint concerns the upper limbs.

Having heard the patient's description of the symptoms, it is usually necessary to probe the history of the presenting complaint in specific areas.

Timing of symptoms

Determining the temporal features of a patient's symptoms is essential to reach a pathological diagnosis:

- onset,
- progression,
- duration,
- recovery,
- frequency.

For example, a patient may present with weakness of one side of the body, suggesting a lesion in the contralateral cerebral hemisphere. Detailed further questioning on the timing of the symptoms may clarify the pathological nature of this lesion (Fig. 1.1).

'Discriminant' questions

If the initial history only partially solves the anatomical diagnosis, the 'shortlist' of potential sites may be reduced by asking the patient direct questions (Table 1.2).

For example, a patient presenting with numbness in both hands and both feet is likely to have a diffuse disorder of all the peripheral sensory nerves of the extremities (**sensory polyneuropathy**). But a similar '**glove-and-stocking**' sensory loss may occasionally be produced by

Table 1.2 Neurological systematic review questions: Has the patient suffered any of the following?

Pain
Headache
Facial, neck, back or limb pain
Disturbance of consciousness
Blackouts, faints, fits*
Altered sleep pattern
Cognitive and affective dysfunction
Memory, language
Depression, irritability
Cranial nerve symptoms
Loss of vision, blurred or double vision*
Hearing, sense of taste and smell
Vertigo, dizziness, giddiness*
'Bulbar' problems (swallowing, articulation of speech)
Limb symptoms
Difficulty in lifting, gripping, fine finger movements; clumsiness
Gait disorder, leg weakness or stiffness, balance problems
Loss of sensation, altered sensation, numbness*
Involuntary movements, incoordination
Sphincter disturbance
Bladder, bowel, sexual dysfunction

*If the patient uses terms like blackouts, fainting, dizziness, giddiness, double vision or numbness, it is worthwhile establishing their exact meaning, as the standard medical usage of the term may not correspond to the patient's intended meaning.

a **cervical spinal cord lesion**, mimicking a polyneuropathy.

In this instance, selecting questions from Table 1.2 likely to *discriminate* between these two anatomical diagnoses, a history of neck pain or injury will strongly favour the diagnosis of cervical cord lesion, as will the presence of sphincter dysfunction. Bladder disturbance is an early feature of spinal cord disease but only occurs in patients with a sensory polyneuropathy if there is a coexistent **autonomic** neuropathy.

Upper limit of symptoms

A useful further refinement in neurological history-taking is to check the '**upper anatomi-**cal limit' of the symptoms. Thus, in a patient presenting with weakness of one leg the anatomical diagnostic range is wide. But specifically asking whether there are equivalent symptoms in the ipsilateral arm immediately narrows this range, the patient then being far more likely to have a **hemiparesis** caused by a lesion on the opposite side of the brain than anything else.

Negative and positive symptoms

A valid distinction may be made between 'negative' and 'positive' neurological symptoms.

Negative symptoms, or loss of particular functions, signify destructive lesions of the nervous system. Thus, a vascular event in one cerebral hemisphere will generally lead to loss of function as indicated, for example, by paralysis of the opposite side of the body.

Conversely, **positive symptoms** are those that suggest an irritative lesion, i.e. an area of abnormal excessive electrical activity in the nervous system. An irritative lesion in one cerebral hemisphere may produce repetitive involuntary (**clonic**) movements of groups of muscles on the opposite side of the body (**partial epilepsy**) rather than paralysis.

Remainder of the history

In neurology, as in other branches of medicine, valuable information, particularly about the pathological diagnosis, can be obtained by asking directly about:

- previous medical history,
- family history,
- social history,
- therapeutic history.

Considering again the patient who presents with glove-and-stocking sensory loss caused by a sensory polyneuropathy:

- **Previous medical history**: A history of diabetes mellitus would be especially relevant, this being a common cause of a sensory polyneuropathy.
- **Family history**: Some causes of a polyneuropathy are inherited.

• **Social history**: Excessive alcohol intake may lead to a sensory polyneuropathy, as may accompanying vitamin deficiencies.

• **Therapeutic history**: Many drugs may cause a polyneuropathy.

Witnesses

Many neurological patients are unable to give a complete account of their symptoms, and information must be sought from family members and other witnesses.

A witness account is especially valuable for patients reporting transient alterations in their state of consciousness. By their very nature, such attacks may prevent the patient from recalling the details of all that occurred. In the acute setting of an unconscious patient in the hospital casualty department, obtaining a history from anyone accompanying the patient is essential.

The need for witnesses also applies to those presenting with progressive **cognitive** impairment in adult life (**dementia**). Indeed, corroboration of such symptoms by a close family member lends weight to this diagnosis. A patient who reports problems of memory and intellect unnoticed by family or colleagues at work may be experiencing the consequences of anxiety or depression ('**pseudodementia**') rather than 'organic' dementia, i.e. associated with a recognized macroscopic or microscopic change in brain structure.

History and examination

In neurology, separating the history and examination is artificial in practice, in the sense that the examination really begins before and during the formal history-taking. Much may be learnt from initial impressions of a patient's:
• gait,
• facial expression,
• handshake,
• speech.

The neurological examination must also be performed in the context of the general physical examination. This applies particularly to the cardiovascular and musculoskeletal systems. The following features are important in assessing vascular disease of the nervous system:
• pulse – rate and rhythm,
• blood pressure,
• murmurs and bruits – cardiac, carotid, cranial or spinal.

In the musculoskeletal system, it is important to examine for skull, spine and joint deformity.

The various components of the neurological examination should be 'screened' in each patient:
• level of consciousness,
• cognitive function,
• speech,
• cranial nerves,
• neck and trunk,
• limbs – motor and sensory examination,
• gait.

The detail required for each part will be dictated by the history. Thus, in many standard outpatient consultations, level of consciousness and cognitive function are screened merely by assessing the patient's ability to give a coherent history. However, in the emergency setting of an unconscious patient in the casualty department, or a confused patient on a general medical ward, these aspects require much more detailed assessment. The remaining chapters of this section outline these parts of the neurological examination in the context of relevant anatomy and physiology.

> **Key points**
>
> • Neurological diagnosis is best divided into two steps: site of lesion (anatomical diagnosis) and disease process (pathological diagnosis).
> • The time course of a patient's symptoms provides clues to the pathological diagnosis.
> • Neurological symptoms may be negative (loss of function) or positive.
> • History from witnesses is essential for patients presenting with disturbances of consciousness, or with cognitive impairment.
> • A full neurological examination is time-consuming and potentially exhausting for patient and doctor; selection of the components requiring detailed assessment is determined by the history.

Chapter 2

Consciousness

Consciousness is an individual's awareness of self and surroundings. This definition is narrow and incomplete but useful in the clinical context of acute disturbances of consciousness. Pathophysiologically, normal consciousness depends on the sensory input into the brain and the intrinsic activity of the reticular activating system, the ascending reticular formation in the brainstem and its rostral connections, which maintain the cerebral cortex in an alert state.

In clinical practice, previous attempts to classify the severity of an alteration in level of consciousness, using imprecise terms such as stupor, semi-coma, have been superseded by the **Glasgow Coma Scale** (Table 2.1).This more objective approach has become universally accepted as valuable in assessing a patient's initial condition and subsequent response to treatment and time.

Causes of altered level of consciousness

The normal function of the reticular activating system may be disturbed by focal structural lesions of the brain or by more diffuse processes:
- Structural
  - infratentorial (directly involving the brainstem) (e.g. trauma, infarction, haemorrhage, tumour, demyelination),

- supratentorial (compressing the brainstem) (similar pathological causes, particularly affecting the right cerebral hemisphere);
- Diffuse
  - decreased availability of substances required for normal brain metabolism (hypoxia, hypoglycaemia),
  - other metabolic disorders (e.g. renal and liver failure, hypothermia, vitamin deficiencies),
  - epilepsy (interfering with the normal electrical activity of the brainstem),
  - inflammation of the brain or its coverings (encephalitis, meningitis),
  - drugs and toxins (opiates, antidepressants, hypnotics, alcohol).

Management of the unconscious patient

The emergency management of the unconscious patient consists first of protecting respiratory and circulatory function with standard life support techniques.

Airway – remove any obstruction, use oropharyngeal airway or endotracheal tube if necessary.

Breathing – give oxygen, ventilate if respiratory movements are inadequate.

Circulation – check pulse and blood pressure, gain intravenous access and replace any blood loss.

Lecture Notes: Neurology, 9th edition. By Lionel Ginsberg. Published 2010 by Blackwell Publishing.

Table 2.1 Glasgow Coma Scale.

	Score
Eye opening	
Spontaneously	4
To speech	3
To pain	2
None	1
Best verbal response	
Orientated	5
Confused	4
Inappropriate words	3
Incomprehensible sounds	2
None	1
Best motor response	
Obeying commands	6
Localizing pain	5
Withdraws (normal flexion)	4
Flexes abnormally (spastic flexion)	3
Extending to pain	2
None	1
TOTAL	3–15

Any immediately reversible cause should be treated:

- Is the patient hypoglycaemic?
  - Administer 50 mL 50% intravenous dextrose.
- Is there evidence of drug overdosage?
  - Administer appropriate antidote: naloxone for opiates; flumazenil for benzodiazepines.

Other treatable causes should be identified from any history available from witnesses or relatives and from the physical examination (looking particularly for evidence of injury, infection, epilepsy (Chapter 10) and raised intracranial pressure (Chapter 13)). After these emergency measures are completed, detailed neurological examination of the eyes (Chapter 4) and limbs may help localize the site of brain damage. The presence of focal neurological signs is more in keeping with structural rather than diffuse metabolic or toxic causes.

Brain death and its differential diagnosis

In some patients, irreversible brain damage may have occurred with permanent destruction of brainstem function and hence death of the patient, yet cardiovascular function may remain stable and respiration be maintained by artificial ventilatory support. In these circumstances, formal criteria of **brainstem death** are used to decide whether cardiorespiratory support should be withdrawn (Table 2.2). This has become an important ethical and practical concern, particularly with the advent of transplantation surgery.

An even more difficult ethical situation arises when patients have preserved brainstem function yet widespread severe brain damage. In one such circumstance, the **vegetative state**, individuals are unaware of self and environment yet able to breathe spontaneously, with a stable circulation and cycles of eye closure and opening resembling sleep and waking. This state may be permanent.

Equally distressing for relatives and carers, and infinitely more so for the patient, is the converse situation where the function of the reticular activating system is preserved despite extensive brainstem damage. The patient is alert but paralysed, able to communicate only by means of blinking and vertical eye movements (**locked-in syndrome**).

Transient disturbance of consciousness

Patients with transient episodes of altered consciousness constitute a common diagnostic problem in neurological outpatient practice. The main differential diagnosis is between **epilepsy** (Chapter 10) and **syncope**.

Syncope is loss of consciousness caused by a transient reduction in blood flow to the brain for which there are many causes:

- cardiac arrhythmias,
- prolonged standing, especially in warm surroundings,
- psychogenic factors, e.g. simple faint in squeamish individuals exposed to needles and other medical procedures,
- other causes of excessive reflex vagal stimulation, e.g. **micturition syncope**, **cough syncope**.

Table 2.2 Criteria for brainstem death.

Preconditions

Central nervous system depressant drugs must not be contributing to the clinical state

The patient must be on a ventilator due to inadequate spontaneous respiration; effects of neuromuscular blocking agents must be excluded

Hypothermia and severe metabolic disorders must not be possible primary causes of the patient's condition

The cause of the patient's condition must be established and must be compatible with irreversible brain damage

Tests

No pupillary response to light

Absent corneal reflexes (Chapter 4)

Absent vestibulo-ocular reflex (see Fig. 4.7)

No gag or response to tracheal suction

No motor response in cranial nerve territory to painful stimulus, e.g. supraorbital pressure

No respiratory movements when patient is disconnected from ventilator (Pao_2 is maintained by passing O_2 at 6 L/min down endotracheal tube; $Paco_2$ should be allowed to rise above 6.65 kPa, 50 mmHg)

Notes

Tests should be carried out by two doctors, both with appropriate expertise and one, preferably both, of consultant status

The tests should be repeated at an interval; death is certified at the time of the second set of tests, assuming no evidence of brainstem function is detected

The EEG (Chapter 8) is of no value in diagnosing brain death

Typically, patients may have a warning before losing consciousness and falling, with lightheadedness, nausea, blurred or tunnel vision, pallor and sweating. Once the patient is in a supine position, with the head at the same level as the heart, recovery is usually rapid (1–2 minutes or less) provided there is no continuing cardiac dysrhythmia. If falling is impeded, brain hypoxia may be prolonged and convulsive movements may occur.

Other important differential diagnoses for epilepsy and syncope are:

- Hypoglycaemia
  - Warning symptoms include anxiety, tremor, unsteadiness, sweating and hunger. Loss of consciousness may be prolonged (1 hour or more) and convulsions may occur.
- Drop attacks
  - In middle-aged and elderly women, falls without warning and without clear-cut loss of consciousness. Though usually of no sinister significance, injuries may occur because of the lack of warning.
- Psychogenic attacks

- Either in stressful situations or as attention-seeking behaviour. These attacks may be associated with **hyperventilation** with tingling in the extremities, and may sometimes be reproduced by voluntary hyperventilation.

Sleep disorders

Sleep is a normal state of altered consciousness dependent on the intrinsic rhythmicity of the reticular activating system (sleep–wake cycle). In contrast to pathological unconsciousness, a sleeping person is easily roused. Certain disorders are characterized by excessive daytime sleep, as follows.

Narcolepsy

This rare disorder consists of a tetrad of clinical features:

- **Daytime sleep attacks** (narcolepsy), typically lasting 10–20 minutes, from which the patient awakes refreshed. These episodes are irresistible and may occur under inappropriate circumstances, e.g. during conversations, meals, driving.

- **Cataplexy**: episodes of loss of postural control and limb weakness with preserved consciousness, often provoked by emotional events, e.g. laughter.
- **Sleep paralysis**: inability to move while falling asleep or waking.
- **Hypnagogic hallucinations**: frightening visual hallucinations on falling asleep.

The cause of the disease is poorly understood, though there may be a genetic basis and an association with the HLA (human leukocyte antigen; major histocompatibility) complex. Narcolepsy may be treated with amphetamines, but in view of the addictive properties of these drugs, care must be taken to reach the correct diagnosis. An alternative newer drug is modafinil. Clomipramine relieves cataplexy but has no effect on narcoleptic attacks. Other antidepressants are also effective against cataplexy.

Obstructive sleep apnoea

An under-recognized cause of excessive daytime somnolence arises in patients with partial upper airways obstruction, where further narrowing or collapse during sleep results in nocturnal apnoeic attacks. These patients generally have a disrupted night's sleep with heavy snoring. They wake unrefreshed and are sleepy during the day, but daytime sleep episodes are also not refreshing. Features of the narcolepsy complex are absent. There may be a history of otolaryngological disease and sometimes an association with obesity and excess alcohol intake. The diagnosis may be reached by recording upper airways obstruction and apnoeic episodes despite continuing respiratory effort using overnight **pulse oximetry** at home or more detailed studies in a sleep laboratory. Detailed sleep studies may be required to exclude the rarer syndrome of **central sleep apnoea**, where apnoeic episodes occur without continuing respiratory effort. Patients with obstructive sleep apnoea may be successfully treated using a device at home to maintain nasal **continuous positive airways pressure** (CPAP) at night and hence prevent collapse of soft tissues which may obstruct the upper airways during sleep. Some patients require surgery to remove excess soft tissue from the upper airways, e.g. nasal polyps, deviated nasal septum, tonsillar hypertrophy.

Key points

- The Glasgow Coma Scale provides an objective measure of a patient's level of consciousness
- Consciousness may be altered as a result of focal structural lesions of the brain, or by more diffuse processes (metabolic, inflammatory, epileptic or toxic)
- The emergency management of an unconscious patient first entails attention to airway, breathing and circulation
- Brainstem death is diagnosed using strict clinical criteria
- The main differential diagnosis in patients presenting with transient disturbances of consciousness lies between epilepsy and syncope

Chapter 3

Cognitive function

Higher brain function may be subclassified into:
- **Distributed functions**, which do not localize to a particular brain region but instead require the concerted action of multiple parts on both sides of the brain, e.g.
  - attention and concentration,
  - memory,
  - higher-order executive function,
  - social conduct and personality;
- **Localized functions**, which are dependent on the normal structure and function of a particular part of one cerebral hemisphere (Fig. 3.1).

Distributed cognitive function

Attention and concentration

Anatomy

The maintenance of normal attention is dependent on the same anatomical basis as that of consciousness, i.e. the reticular activating system which projects to the thalamus and then to the cerebral cortex diffusely.

Examination

Clinical tests of attention and concentration include:
- **Orientation** in time and place – Can the patient state the time of day, day of the week, the correct month and year, and the name of the building where they are?
- **Digit span** – ability to repeat a list of digits forwards and backwards.
- **'Serial sevens'** – ability to subtract seven repeatedly starting from 100, or, failing this, to count backwards from 20 or recite the months of the year backwards.

Clinical aspects

The syndrome most associated with impaired attention and concentration is the **acute confusional state**, nowadays usually called **delirium**, or sometimes **acute organic brain syndrome**, a very common management problem in general medicine, particularly in the elderly. Other features of this state include:
- muddled thinking and hence speech,
- visual hallucinations,
- disturbed sleep–wake cycle, the patient often being awake and indeed more confused at night,
- memory impairment – with an inability to register new material,
- mood changes.

Lecture Notes: Neurology, 9th edition. By Lionel Ginsberg. Published 2010 by Blackwell Publishing.

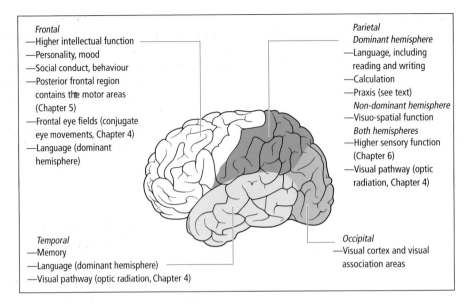

Frontal
—Higher intellectual function
—Personality, mood
—Social conduct, behaviour
—Posterior frontal region
  contains the motor areas
  (Chapter 5)
—Frontal eye fields (conjugate
  eye movements, Chapter 4)
—Language (dominant
  hemisphere)

Parietal
Dominant hemisphere
—Language, including
  reading and writing
—Calculation
—Praxis (see text)
Non-dominant hemisphere
—Visuo-spatial function
Both hemispheres
—Higher sensory function
  (Chapter 6)
—Visual pathway (optic
  radiation, Chapter 4)

Temporal
—Memory
—Language (dominant hemisphere)
—Visual pathway (optic radiation, Chapter 4)

Occipital
—Visual cortex and visual
  association areas

Figure 3.1 Functional localization in the lobes of the brain.

The patient may be restless and excitable, or alternatively subdued and apathetic.

As might be predicted from the anatomy, the causes of delirium are the same as those of an altered level of consciousness (Chapter 2). Indeed, it may be regarded as the mild end of a spectrum which proceeds in severity to coma. Depending on the cause, the state is usually transient, typically lasting a few days.

Memory

Definitions

The memory 'system' has been subdivided into multiple components:
• **Implicit memory**. Learned motor responses not available to conscious access, e.g. driving a car and other complex motor skills.
• **Explicit memory**. Available to conscious access, further subclassified as:
  • **episodic memory**, e.g. recalling autobiographical details and other personally experienced events relating to specific times;
  • **semantic memory** – general store of world knowledge.

Other useful concepts are as follows:
• **Short-term memory** – working memory responsible for **immediate** recall of small amounts of verbal or spatial material.
• **Anterograde memory** – acquisition of new material.
• **Retrograde memory** – recall of previously learnt information.

Anatomy

The anatomical basis for episodic memory is the **limbic system** (including the hippocampus and thalamus and their connections), whereas semantic memory relies on the **temporal neocortex**. Implicit memory involves various structures, including the basal ganglia and cerebellum and their connections with the cerebral cortex.

Examination

Bedside tests of memory function include:
• recall of complex verbal information (a name and address after 5–10 min, lists of words, stories) and geometric figures – for verbal and non-verbal anterograde episodic memory, respectively,

Table 3.1 Classification of amnesia.

	Acute, transient	Chronic, persistent
Isolated	Transient global amnesia	Amnesic syndrome
With other cognitive deficits	Delirium	Dementia

- recall of autobiographical details – for retrograde episodic memory,
- tests of general knowledge and vocabulary – for semantic memory, e.g. recent news items, names of political and other world figures.

Clinical aspects

Amnesia may be acute and transient, or chronic and persistent. It may occur in relative isolation or in the context of other cognitive deficits (Table 3.1).

Transient global amnesia is a condition in which a middle-aged or elderly patient suddenly becomes profoundly amnesic with loss of both anterograde and retrograde memory. The latter may stretch back months or years. The patient seems bewildered, repetitively asking simple questions ('What happened?'), but without impairment of consciousness or other cognitive deficits. Recovery occurs within a few hours, including the retrograde amnesia, so that the patient is ultimately only left with amnesia for the period of the attack. Recurrence is rare and the prognosis is good. Previously thought to be a manifestation of cerebrovascular disease, the cause remains unknown, though there is an association with migraine.

Some patients with recurrent episodes have epilepsy of temporal lobe origin (Chapter 10) – 'transient epileptic amnesia'. These episodes are typically briefer than those of transient global amnesia, usually lasting less than 1 hour.

The **amnesic syndrome** refers to chronic and persistent memory failure (anterograde and retrograde), usually irreversible, but again with sparing of other cognitive functions. It is caused by fo-

cal damage to the limbic system, e.g. hippocampal anoxia, damage to the hippocampus from herpes simplex virus encephalitis (Chapter 14), thalamic infarction, vitamin B_1 deficiency (**Korsakoff's syndrome** – Chapter 19) and closed head injury. Severe amnesia is also typically the earliest feature of Alzheimer's disease (Chapter 18).

Amnesia occurs acutely and transiently in the presence of other cognitive deficits in delirium and persistently with other such deficits in **dementia** (see below).

Higher-order executive function, personality and behaviour

Executive function is difficult to define precisely, but involves ability to plan, adapt, handle abstract concepts and solve problems, coupled with aspects of social behaviour and personality, e.g. initiative, motivation and inhibition.

Anatomy

The frontal lobes of the cerebral hemispheres, particularly the **prefrontal areas**, are essential for normal executive function while the ventromedial frontal lobes play a crucial role in social cognition, personality and behaviour.

Examination

Tests of frontal lobe dysfunction are relatively crude and more information may be obtained from the history of informants, e.g. family members (Can the patient hold down a job? Go shopping?) and from clinical observation.

Patients with bifrontal dysfunction may perform poorly on tests of:
- **verbal fluency**, e.g. listing items that can be bought in a supermarket, words beginning with a particular letter;
- **proverb interpretation** – giving concrete explanations of their meaning;
- **cognitive estimates**, e.g. estimating the height of a well-known building.

Perseveration is also a feature of frontal lobe damage – compulsive repetition of words or movements.

With more severe frontal lobe damage, there is loss of **inhibitory control**: patients may become irritable and aggressive, with a decline in social behaviour and hygiene, leading ultimately to incontinence. Whereas some patients are jocular and noisy, others are more passive, speaking and moving little, in extreme instances reaching a state of **akinetic mutism**.

Loss of normal frontal lobe inhibition may result in the appearance of **primitive reflexes**, of which the two most useful are:

• **grasping** – involuntary grasp elicited by stroking the patient's palm, more significant if the patient is distracted at the time, and indicating disease of the contralateral frontal lobe;

• **pouting** – elicited by tapping a spatula placed on the patient's lips, which, if the sign is positive, pucker towards the spatula. In extreme instances, a patient may suck an object presented to their lips.

Clinical aspects

Frontal lobe damage may result from trauma, tumours, infarction and focal degenerative diseases.

Localized cognitive function

Hemisphere dominance

In most individuals, the left cerebral hemisphere is dominant for language function. Even the majority of left-handed people are left hemisphere dominant.

Dominant hemisphere function

Language

Definitions

Aphasia or **dysphasia** is impairment of language function as a result of brain damage. This includes both the spoken word and reading and writing, which may be impaired selectively (**alexia/dyslexia** and **agraphia/dysgraphia**, respectively).

Dysphasia must be distinguished from **dysarthria**, which is impairment of **articulation**, as a result of disease of the muscles involved in speech or their innervation (including lower ('**bulbar'**) cranial nerves, brainstem, cerebellum, basal ganglia and cerebral hemispheres). **Mutism** is complete failure of speech output, which may arise from severe dysphasia or dysarthria (anarthria), or may signify psychiatric disease.

Examination

Clinical tests of language function include:

• **Fluency** – Can the patient produce phrases of normal length (five or more words) in spontaneous speech? If speech is non-fluent, grammar (syntax) is usually abnormal.

• **Comprehension** – Can the patient point on command to everyday objects arranged in front of them, e.g. pen, watch, keys? Can they obey more complex commands? ('You pick up the keys and give me the pen.') Can they understand conceptually based questions? ('What do you call the thin grey dust left after smoking a cigarette?')

• **Repetition** – Can the patient repeat single words or whole sentences such as 'No ifs, ands, or buts'?

• **Naming**, e.g. of everyday items, such as a watch, pen and less familiar objects – nib, buckle, winder (naming objects is impaired (**anomia**) in all dysphasic patients to some extent).

In addition, reading and writing may be tested separately.

Clinical anatomy

Using these bedside tests, a dysphasic patient's language function may be subclassified and localized more accurately in the dominant hemisphere (Fig. 3.2). Focal damage to the different language areas may be due to trauma, infarction or tumour. Writing ability localizes in the region of the **angular gyrus** which is posterior to the major language areas. Lesions in this region, in addition to causing dysgraphia, classically produce other deficits, including **dyscalculia** – impaired number

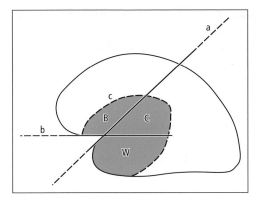

Figure 3.2 Localization and subclassification of dysphasic syndromes. Lesions anterior to line 'a', through the central sulcus of the dominant hemisphere, produce non-fluent dysphasia. Posteriorly, fluency is retained. Below line 'b', through the Sylvian fissure, comprehension is affected; above this line, it is spared. Lesions within the domain circumscribed by line 'c' affect the patient's ability to repeat phrases; outside this line, repetition is preserved. Thus, Broca's aphasia (B) is non-fluent; repetition is affected but comprehension relatively spared. The diagram works equally well for conduction aphasia (C) and Wernicke's aphasia (W). Global aphasia affects all aspects of language function.

comprehension and writing, and hence calculating ability.

Praxis

Dyspraxia is the inability to perform complex motor acts despite normal muscle power, sensation and coordination, and good comprehension and cooperation. It may be tested by asking the patient to copy gestures or to mime the use of imagined household items (e.g., hammer, scissors). Damage to the dominant parietal lobe may result in dyspraxia. Pathways for normal praxis pass from this region to the ipsilateral premotor area in the frontal lobe, and to the equivalent region in the other hemisphere via the corpus callosum.

Non-dominant hemisphere function

Whereas most language function resides in the dominant hemisphere, the non-dominant hemi-sphere is largely, though not exclusively, responsible for **visuo-spatial** skills.

Neglect

Patients with an acute extensive right hemisphere lesion, e.g. a stroke, may behave as though the left half of the world has ceased to exist. This may apply to the patient's own body and to extrapersonal space. Thus, they may:

- deny disability of the left side of the body, even if it has been paralysed by the stroke,
- claim that their left arm belongs to somebody else,
- ignore visual and tactile stimuli presented to the left side,
- dress only the right side, eat food only from the right side of a plate.

Neglect may be tested clinically by asking the patient to copy a drawing of a house or clock face – the left side will be omitted. More subtle abnormalities may be detected by asking the patient to cross out an array of letters on a page, or to bisect lines of varying length (neglect patients consistently bisect to the right of the mid-point).

The mechanisms underlying neglect remain controversial, but it is an important and under-recognized phenomenon. Although many stroke patients recover from neglect, some have persistent problems, profoundly hindering their rehabilitation.

Dressing 'apraxia'

Patients with right-sided hemisphere lesions are often unable to dress properly. The term 'apraxia' is used incorrectly in this context, as the problem is not motor but rather visuo-spatial, relating the orientation of body parts to clothing.

Constructional 'apraxia'

Non-dominant parietal lesions are particularly likely to affect ability to copy complex shapes, e.g. a cube, star or intersecting pentagons. Again, the term 'apraxia' is inappropriate, as the task is largely visuo-spatial rather than primarily motor.

Agnosias

More complex visuo-perceptual disorders usually denote bilateral parieto-occipitotemporal damage and include:

- inability to recognize objects presented visually (**visual object agnosia**) – this disorder can only be diagnosed provided there is no dysphasia, basic visual dysfunction or general intellectual underfunctioning,
- inability to recognize familiar faces (**prosopagnosia**),
- central defects of colour vision.

Dementia

Dementia may be defined as acquired global impairment of intellectual function, usually progressive, and occurring in a setting of clear consciousness. More precisely, a demented patient has significant impairment of two or more areas of cognition (one of which must be memory, the other domains being language, praxis, visuo-spatial skills, personality, social behaviour or abstract thought) in the absence of delirium and of psychiatric disease, such as depression or schizophrenia, which may mimic dementia. Causes of dementia are given in Chapter 18.

Cortical and subcortical dementia

A useful subdivision of dementias is between those where the cerebral cortex is the primary site of disease and those with major involvement of subcortical structures (though some disorders present a mixed picture). In cortical dementias, patients have impaired memory, language, praxis and/or visuo-spatial function. Subcortical dementias are more characterized by slowing of cognitive function (**bradyphrenia**) and by personality and mood disturbances. Patients appear apathetic and

inert, with other features of frontal dysfunction. Though memory is affected, language, praxis and visuo-spatial skills are relatively spared, at least initially.

Neuropsychological evaluation

Distributed and localized cognitive function may be assessed clinically using the various components of the examination outlined briefly in this chapter. In addition, there are standardized **mental test schedules** such as the **mini-mental state examination** (MMSE). This 30-point test includes questions which assess orientation, attention, memory, language and visuo-spatial function. A score below 24/30 on this test is suggestive of dementia. However, this overall test score is insensitive to early dementia, particularly if premorbid intellectual ability was superior, and to circumscribed cognitive deficits, especially those involving non-dominant hemisphere and frontal lobe function. Furthermore, owing to changes in copyright, use of the MMSE is now restricted. Many patients with cognitive deficits require more detailed psychometric evaluation by a neuropsychologist.

Key points

- Cognitive function may be subclassified as distributed or localized (to a particular part of the brain)
- The hallmark of delirium is impaired attention and concentration
- Persistent memory failure may occur in isolation (amnesic syndrome) or in association with other cognitive deficits (dementia)
- Dysphasia is impairment of language function due to brain damage
- The non-dominant hemisphere is largely responsible for visuo-spatial skills

Chapter 4

Vision and other cranial nerves

The human brain is highly adapted for processing visual information. The topical diagnosis of dysfunction in the anterior visual pathways and ocular motility disorders depends upon careful neuro-ophthalmological examination involving the upper cranial nerves. The lower cranial nerves, emerging from the medulla oblongata ('**bulbar nerves**'), form a separate group, concerned primarily with articulation of speech and swallowing.

I: Olfactory nerve

In a routine cranial nerve examination, it is sufficient simply to ask whether the patient has been aware of any deterioration in sense of smell. If the history indicates the need for more detailed assessment, each nostril should be tested individually with bottles containing various aromatic oils (e.g., lavender, peppermint). It is more important for the patient to be able to detect different odours than to name them accurately. Care must be taken to distinguish between substances stimulating the olfactory nerves, and more pungent, irritant chemicals, e.g. ammonia, detected via trigeminal nerve endings in the nasal mucosa. Patients who have lost their sense of smell (**anosmia**) will still respond to ammonia, via this alternative pathway.

Anosmia, particularly if unilateral, may indicate the presence of a tumour involving the olfactory groove (such tumours may also affect vision – Chapter 13). However, more common causes of anosmia include recurrent upper respiratory infections damaging the olfactory mucosa (with smoking as a further contributory factor), head injury (with shearing of olfactory neurones as they pass centrally through the cribriform plate of the ethmoid bone) and neurodegenerative disorders, particularly Parkinson's disease.

The olfactory pathways may give rise to positive, as well as negative, clinical features, in their most extreme form **olfactory hallucinations**, as occur in epilepsy of temporal lobe origin (Chapter 10).

II: Optic nerve

The clinical assessment of the optic nerve involves five components:
- visual acuity,
- visual fields,
- colour vision,
- fundoscopy,
- pupillary responses.

Visual acuity

This is best examined with a **Snellen chart**, the patient reading the lines of letters from a distance

Lecture Notes: Neurology, 9th edition. By Lionel Ginsberg. Published 2010 by Blackwell Publishing.

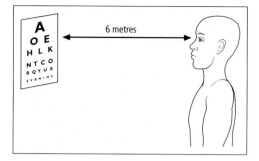

Figure 4.1 Visual acuity testing with the Snellen chart.

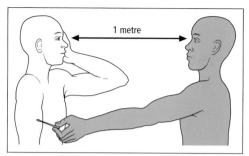

Figure 4.2 Visual field testing by confrontation.

of 6 m (20 feet in the United States) (Fig. 4.1). Each eye is tested individually, and refractive errors are corrected either with lenses or by looking through a pinhole. Acuity is expressed as a fraction, the numerator being the distance between patient and chart, and the denominator being given by the line of letters of smallest size the patient can read accurately. Thus, 6/6 (or 20/20 in the United States – both fractions can be expressed as a decimal acuity of 1.0) is normal, whereas 6/60 (20/200; 0.1) indicates the patient is only able to read the largest letter at the top of the chart. If this letter cannot be read, the chart can be brought closer, or the ability of the patient to count fingers, detect hand movements or to perceive light at all assessed (recorded as CF, HM and PL, respectively). Near vision charts, which involve reading print of varying size, are primarily useful in assessing the need for near correction but are a valuable additional test, particularly in patients with visual field defects who may find it difficult to locate the letters on a distance chart. Visual acuity is impaired early in diseases of the optic nerve and in retinal conditions involving the macula.

Visual fields

The patient's field of vision may be tested at the bedside by **confrontation**. An object is moved tangentially to or from the centre of the visual field (each eye tested individually) in each of the four quadrants (Fig. 4.2). The patient fixes vision on the examiner's pupil and reports the limits of per-

ception of the moving object. A red pin is useful for assessing small areas of defective vision (**scotomas**), caused by retinal disease or optic neuropathy. Relative scotomas can be detected when the target does not disappear completely but the colour is lost. Lesions posterior to the optic chiasm are often detectable with much larger stimuli, e.g. a moving finger, or the ability to count fingers in the four quadrants of vision.

Nerve fibres in the visual pathways retain a crude spatial relationship to each other, reflecting their origin in the retina. This fact and the partial decussation of the pathways at the optic chiasm produce characteristic patterns of visual field disturbance, which greatly aid in lesion localization (Fig. 4.3).

In addition to the classical hemianopias and quadrantanopias, other important field defects and related phenomena detectable at the bedside include:

• **Central scotoma** – loss of central vision generally associated with a reduction in visual acuity, and characteristic of diseases of the optic nerve and the macular region of the retina.

• Enlargement of the **physiological blind spot**, seen with swelling of the optic disc (**papilloedema**) caused by raised intracranial pressure (Chapters 9 and 13), and typically occurring with preserved visual acuity.

• **Macular sparing** – preservation of the macular (central) region in patients with a homonymous hemianopia (Fig. 4.3) may be due to a lesion of the visual cortex sparing the occipital pole where the macular region is represented.

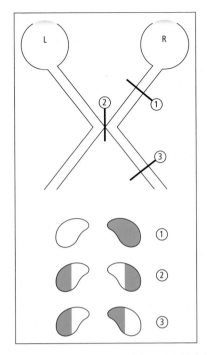

Figure 4.3 Anatomical localization of visual field defects. (1) Lesions of the optic nerve produce monocular visual loss. (2) A lesion of the optic chiasm typically damages the decussating fibres from the nasal halves of the retinae, resulting in a **bitemporal hemianopia** (light from the temporal half-field of vision is received and processed by the nasal part of the retina). (3) An optic tract lesion produces a **homonymous hemianopia**. Fibres from the temporal half of one retina are damaged alongside decussated fibres from the nasal half of the other retina. Visual fields are recorded by convention as if the patient is looking at the page. Lesions posterior to the optic tract produce variants of a homonymous hemianopia (though sometimes with **macular sparing** – see text). The spatial relationship of the nerve fibres is preserved even in the posterior parts of the visual pathways. Thus, a parietal lobe lesion will damage the superior fibres of the optic radiation, resulting in an inferior **homonymous quadrantanopia**. Conversely, a temporal lobe lesion will produce a superior homonymous quadrantanopia. Note that superior and inferior are reversed along with nasal and temporal, throughout the visual pathway. The retinal representation is rotated 180° compared to the actual object being viewed, as in a camera.

- **Tunnel vision** – loss of the peripheral fields with preservation of the central region arises for several reasons:
  - ophthalmological disease – chronic simple glaucoma,

- retinal disease – retinitis pigmentosa,
- cortical disease – bilateral homonymous hemi-anopias with macular sparing.

Commonly, however, it is a 'functional' or simulated phenomenon (Chapter 19) in patients with no neurological or ophthalmological disease. In this case, the preserved visual field may not expand at increasing viewing distances, as would be expected from the laws of geometry.

- **Visual inattention** – may be detected by simultaneously presenting a patient with stimuli in both visual half-fields, when the patient has both eyes open. The stimulus contralateral to a diseased cerebral hemisphere (usually the non-dominant) may be missed, even in subtle parieto-occipital lesions that are not gross enough to produce a hemianopic field defect.

Most visual field abnormalities can be assessed by confrontation at the bedside. Occasionally, however, a more carefully defined stimulus (in terms of size and colour) and map of the visual fields (e.g., using a tangent [Bjerrum] screen, bowl perimeter [Goldmann] or automated [Humphrey] equipment) are necessary. These techniques are particularly valuable for small scotomas, e.g. caused by retinal disease, and to monitor a patient's progress with time and therapy.

Colour vision

Clinical testing of colour vision usually involves the **Ishihara plates**. These consist of coloured dots arranged such that individuals with normal colour vision can read a number 'hidden' in the pattern of the dots. Defective colour vision may be inherited as a sex-linked recessive trait. It may also be acquired, particularly in optic nerve disorders. Thus, **desaturation** of colour (especially red) vision is an early feature of all optic nerve disease. More subtle central (i.e. cerebral) defects of colour vision, usually caused by occipitotemporal disease, and often involving both hemispheres, may require more sophisticated testing.

Fundoscopy

The prime use of the ophthalmoscope in neurological practice is for inspection of the optic disc (Fig. 4.4a). Two major patterns of abnormality are detectable:

- **Optic atrophy** (Fig. 4.4b) – pallor of the optic nerve head because of atrophy of the fibres (causes summarized in Table 4.1).
- **Swelling of the optic disc** (Fig. 4.4c), sometimes with surrounding (**peripapillary**) haemorrhage or haemorrhage on the disc itself. This appearance may develop in two different pathological circumstances:
  - raised intracranial pressure transmitted to the optic nerve sheath, resulting in bilateral **papilloedema**;
  - local inflammatory processes involving the optic nerve near the retina (optic neuritis).

These two possibilities are generally readily distinguished by assessment of the visual acuity. In papilloedema, acuity is preserved until late, whereas in optic neuritis there is early loss of acuity in association with a central scotoma. Furthermore, optic neuritis is usually unilateral.

Other uses of the ophthalmoscope in neurology include detection of the effects of general medical conditions that may also have neurological consequences (e.g., diabetes, hypertension) and of ophthalmological disorders that may be associated with neurological disease, e.g. retinitis pigmentosa.

Pupillary reactions

Anatomy

The afferent component of the reflex arc by which the pupils constrict in response to light, or to **accommodation** for near vision, is conveyed initially by the optic nerve. The efferent nerves are part of the parasympathetic nervous system (Chapter 7), and reach the pupilloconstrictor smooth muscle fibres (sphincter pupillae) via the third (oculomotor) nerve. Pupillodilator muscle fibres are supplied by sympathetic nerves, which reach the eye (from the superior cervical ganglion)

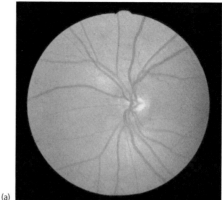

(a)

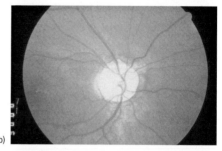

(b)

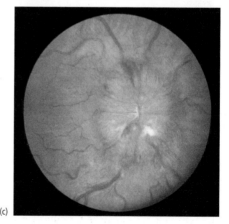

(c)

Figure 4.4 Fundoscopic appearances of the optic disc. (a) Normal; (b) optic atrophy; (c) swollen haemorrhagic disc – papilloedema. Note that bilateral papilloedema does not necessarily signify an intracranial mass lesion. Intracranial pressure may rise for other reasons, including systemic hypertension, benign (idiopathic) intracranial hypertension (Chapter 9), meningitis, subarachnoid haemorrhage, intracranial venous sinus thrombosis (Chapter 11) and carbon dioxide retention. Furthermore, similar appearances of the optic disc may be seen with anaemia and polycythaemia and in circumstances where the CSF protein concentration is very high.

Table 4.1 Causes of optic atrophy.

Inherited
Leber's hereditary optic neuropathy (Chapter 18)
Hereditary ataxias
Acquired
Trauma (e.g., orbital fracture or indirect trauma)
Infection/inflammation
Optic neuritis (e.g., in multiple sclerosis)
Syphilis, sarcoidosis
Spread (e.g., from sinuses)
Tumour
Direct compression of anterior visual pathway (e.g., tumour of optic nerve, pituitary or sphenoid)
Following long-standing papilloedema ('secondary optic atrophy')
Vascular
Compression by carotid aneurysm
Ischaemic optic neuropathy
Toxic/metabolic (disc may appear normal) (e.g., diabetes, methanol, tobacco, ethambutol, vitamin B_{12} deficiency)
Optic atrophy may also result from ophthalmological disease
Raised intraocular pressure (glaucoma)
Retinal disorders (e.g., macular degeneration, retinitis pigmentosa)

via the sympathetic plexus on the wall of the internal carotid artery.

Examination

The pupils are first inspected for:

• Size – recording the diameter in millimetres and bearing in mind that many drugs can affect pupil size, e.g. anticholinergic agents instilled topically to dilate the pupil for ophthalmoscopic inspection of the retina, pinpoint pupils caused by opiate overdosage. Size should be recorded at three ambient light levels: high, intermediate and low. Many normal individuals have pupils that are unequal in size (**physiological anisocoria**); in this case the difference will be the same at all light levels.

• Shape – the normal circular shape of the pupil may be disrupted by trauma, both accidental and surgical, and segmental denervation. Local inflammatory disease (iritis) may also render the pupil irregular in shape as a result of adhesions (**synechiae**) between the iris and structures behind it.

• Eccentricity – the pupil may deviate from its normal central location as a result of trauma.

Once these observations have been made on the resting pupils, their response to light and accommodation should be tested. Shining a bright light, e.g. from a pen torch, abruptly into one pupil normally produces a brisk constriction on that side and a simultaneous identical response in the other eye (**direct** and **consensual** light reflexes, respectively). The pupils also normally constrict when a subject shifts focus from the distance to a near object. In older individuals, when the lens is no longer able to accommodate (i.e., alter its thickness for near and far objects), pupillary constriction still accompanies the convergence of the eyes induced by focusing on a near object.

Disorders of pupillary function

Lesions of the pupillary pathways may be broadly classified into afferent and efferent defects (Fig. 4.5). Afferent defects are often incomplete, i.e. an affected eye may still be able to respond directly to light, but not as well as the other side. Such a **relative afferent pupillary defect** is an important sign of optic neuritis (Chapter 16). It is best demonstrated using the **swinging torch** test, in which light is repeatedly shone into the affected eye alternating with the good side. When the light is shining on the unaffected eye, both pupils constrict. When it is transferred to the diseased eye, there is bilateral pupillary dilatation. This is because the weak direct reflex on the diseased side is more than counterbalanced by the withdrawal of the stimulus from the normal eye, resulting in consensual dilatation.

Abnormalities of pupil size and reactions are frequently encountered in combination with disorders of eye and eyelid movement (see below).

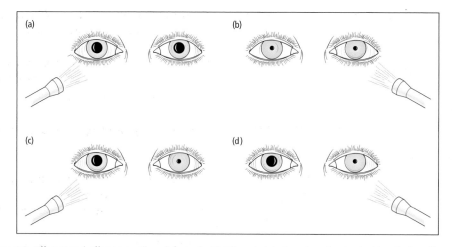

Figure 4.5 Afferent and efferent pupillary defects. (a, b) Afferent defect – when the torch shines in the affected eye (a), light is not perceived and neither pupil constricts. When the normal eye is tested (b), its pupil constricts, as does the other pupil consensually. (c, d) Efferent defect – light is perceived by the affected eye but the pupil cannot respond (c). The other pupil constricts consensually. When the torch shines in the unaffected eye (d), there is direct pupillary constriction but no consensual response from the affected eye.

There are also two well-known pupillary syndromes:

- **Argyll Robertson pupil** – this classical sign of neurosyphilis (and occasionally other disorders) is now rarely seen. The pupil is small and irregular with a preserved near response but reduced or absent light reflex. The condition is usually bilateral.
- **Myotonic pupil** – the affected pupil is dilated, with an impaired response to light but constricts very slowly for near vision. The near response may be tonic, showing delayed redilatation. The condition is benign, may become bilateral and may be associated with absent tendon reflexes (Holmes–Adie syndrome).

III, IV and VI: Oculomotor, trochlear and abducens nerves

Anatomy

The actions of the extraocular muscles are summarized in Fig. 4.6. The superior oblique muscle is supplied by the fourth (trochlear) cranial nerve; lateral rectus by the abducens nerve. All the other muscles are innervated by the oculomotor nerve, which also carries the parasympathetic fibres to the sphincter pupillae, and the nerve

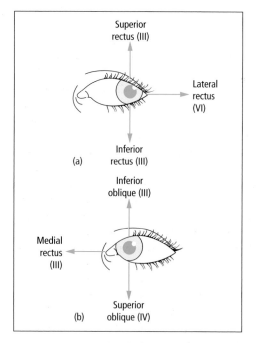

Figure 4.6 Actions and innervation of the extraocular muscles (left eye). When the eye is abducted (a), the superior and inferior rectus muscles are responsible for elevating and depressing the eyeball, respectively. In adduction (b), these actions are taken by the inferior and superior oblique muscles, respectively.

supply to levator palpebrae superioris, the muscle responsible for elevating the eyelid.

Examination

Clinical testing of eye movements in a conscious patient usually involves the subject tracking a moving target (e.g., the physician's finger) in the vertical and horizontal directions. The target should inscribe the shape of the letter H in the air, rather than a simple cross, movements in the vertical direction thereby being examined with the eyes both adducted and abducted. This allows each extraocular muscle to be assessed relatively independently (Fig. 4.6).

Pursuit eye movements tested in this way are the best rapid screening test for disease, as normal pursuit implies the integrity of virtually all the neural pathways involved in the control of eye movement. Parts of this complex system may be examined in relative isolation using alternative clinical methods:

- **Saccades** – these rapid shifts in the position of gaze may be assessed by asking the patient to look swiftly right and left, up and down.
- **Vergence** – the ability of the eyes to converge for near vision, unlike normal pursuit and saccadic movements, where the eyes move in the same direction (**conjugate gaze**).
- **Optokinetic movements** – observed when a cylinder with alternating black and white stripes is rotated in front of the subject's eyes. Normally, slow tracking eye movements are seen to alternate with fast corrective saccades (**optokinetic nystagmus**). Such movements are lost in an unconscious patient. The optokinetic drum is therefore a useful instrument for detecting simulated disturbances of consciousness (Chapter 19).
- **Vestibulo-ocular reflex** – none of the above methods can be used in an unconscious patient. In such instances, brainstem pathways, particularly those connecting the vestibular nuclei (which receive their input from the balance apparatus of the inner ear – see below) to the III, IV and VI nuclei, can still be assessed by:
  - response to head movement (**oculocephalic** or **doll's head reflex**),

  - response to instillation of ice-cold water into the external auditory meatus (**caloric test**) (Fig. 4.7).

These tests are important in the distinction between brainstem function and brainstem death in an unconscious patient (Chapter 2).

Disorders of eye and eyelid movement

Symptoms

Patients may be aware of weakness of levator palpebrae superioris from a tendency for the eyelid to droop or close completely (partial and complete **ptosis**).

Diplopia or double vision in neurological practice arises from malalignment of the eyes such that light from an object falls on non-corresponding sites on the two retinae, and the brain is unable to fuse the resultant images. This **binocular** diplopia, present only when both eyes are open, must be distinguished from **monocular** diplopia, which persists when one eye is covered. The latter is not generally a symptom of neurological disease but occurs in ophthalmological disorders such as lens opacities and is more commonly a 'functional' phenomenon (Chapter 19).

Binocular diplopia arises from an imbalance between the extraocular muscles of the two eyes or of their innervation. It is always sudden in onset (either one has double vision or one does not), but it can vary in severity. Patients may be able to report whether there is horizontal, vertical or oblique separation of the images and whether or not there is torsion of one image.

Syndromes

Abnormalities of eye and eyelid movement in conscious patients are best diagnosed by first determining whether one of the classical patterns of disease is present on inspection and simple pursuit testing, as follows.

Third nerve palsy

In its complete form, there is ptosis, caused by paralysis of levator palpebrae superioris. When the examiner raises the eyelid, the affected eye is seen

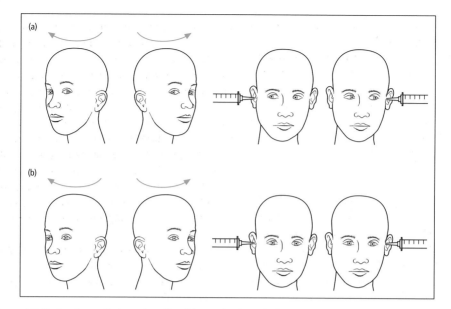

Figure 4.7 Testing the vestibulo-ocular reflex. (a) Intact brainstem – head rotation produces transient eye movement in the opposite direction – oculocephalic or doll's head reflex. Note this reflex also applies to vertical eye movements in response to neck flexion/extension. Caloric testing – instillation of 50 mL iced water into the external auditory meatus produces conjugate deviation of the eyes towards the stimulus. (b) Brainstem death – absent oculocephalic and caloric responses.

in a 'down-and-out' position as a result of the unopposed action of the superior oblique and lateral rectus muscles. A third nerve palsy may also involve the parasympathetic pupillary fibres; hence, the pupil is 'fixed' (no reflex responses) and dilated ('**surgical**' third nerve palsy), but sometimes the pupil is spared ('**medical**' third nerve palsy). Causes of a third nerve palsy are listed in Table 4.2.

Fourth nerve palsy

Isolated unilateral paralysis of the superior oblique muscle may result from minor head trauma. The patient is typically aware of diplopia descending stairs, and may hold the head tilted towards the normal side, in an attempt to correct for the muscle weakness. Superior oblique paralysis may be confirmed by **cover testing** (see below).

Sixth nerve palsy

The patient is unable to abduct the affected eye, in extreme cases resulting in the appearance of a convergent squint at rest, because of the unopposed action of medial rectus. There is diplopia on

Table 4.2 Causes of a third nerve palsy.

Compression
Within brainstem (tumour, basilar aneurysm)
Tentorial herniation (with deteriorating conscious level – 'coning', Chapter 13)
Posterior communicating artery aneurysm
In the cavernous sinus (tumour, aneurysm, thrombosis)
Superior orbital fissure/orbit (tumour, granuloma)
Infarction
In the brainstem
In the nerve trunk – 'medical' causes (diabetes, hypertension, giant cell arteritis, lupus, polyarteritis nodosa)
The nerve may also be involved when there is inflammation or infiltration of the basal meninges (tuberculosis, syphilis, sarcoidosis, carcinoma, lymphoma)

looking to the affected side, with horizontal separation of the images. An isolated sixth nerve palsy is often attributed to damage to the nerve's blood supply (**vasa nervorum**) secondary to diabetes or hypertension. Such **microvascular** events resolve, usually completely, within months. A sixth nerve palsy may also be a **false localizing sign** of raised intracranial pressure (Chapters 9 and 13). This is because the nerve has a long and tortuous intracranial course. Thus, it is vulnerable to the general effects of increased pressure, arising from an intracranial mass which need not necessarily directly compress the nerve.

Horner's syndrome

Part of the muscle responsible for elevating the eyelid is supplied by sympathetic nerve fibres. Thus, a lesion of the superior part of the sympathetic nervous system will result in partial ptosis, in combination with **miosis** (pupillary constriction caused by paralysis of sympathetic pupillodilator fibres). Other, less common, features of Horner's syndrome are that the eye itself may appear withdrawn into the orbit (**enophthalmos**) and there may be reduced or absent sweating (**anhidrosis**) on the affected side of the face. The sympathetic nerve supply to the eye originates in the hypothalamus. A lesion anywhere along its course may result in Horner's syndrome (Fig. 4.8).

Nystagmus

Nystagmus is an involuntary rhythmic oscillatory movement of the eyes, which may be present on attempted sustained horizontal or vertical gaze, or sometimes in the primary position. The 'to-and-fro' movements may be of equal velocity (**pendular nystagmus**), but frequently a slow phase in one direction (drifting back to the primary position from the direction of attempted gaze) alternates with a fast corrective phase in the opposite direction (**jerk nystagmus**). Paradoxically, such nystagmus is defined as 'beating' in the direction of the fast phase, though this is merely a normal saccade attempting to compensate for the pathological process represented by the slow component. Jerk nystagmus may be further classified as:

1° – present only with the eyes looking in the direction of the fast component,

2° – persisting in the primary position of gaze (straight ahead),

3° – present even with the eyes looking in the direction of the slow component.

Nystagmus may be congenital, in which case it is usually pendular. Acquired nystagmus may signify disease of the inner ear (labyrinth) (see below), brainstem or cerebellum, or may arise as a side effect of medication such as anti-epilepsy drugs. Rotatory nystagmus implies a lesion of the vestibular system, either peripheral (labyrinthine) or central (brainstem). Vertical nystagmus, if not drug-induced, usually indicates brainstem disease and has particular localizing value (to the region of the foramen magnum) if down-beating on downgaze. Patients are generally unaware of their nystagmus, though they may have associated vertigo (see below). Occasionally, however, the to-and-fro movements of the eyes are symptomatic (**oscillopsia**), especially with vertical nystagmus, the patient being unpleasantly aware of the surroundings appearing to move up and down.

Internuclear ophthalmoplegia

Normal conjugate gaze to the left or right relies on the lateral rectus muscle of one eye contracting synchronously with the medial rectus of the other. The anatomical basis for this coupling resides in the **medial longitudinal fasciculus**, a bundle of rapidly conducting myelinated nerve fibres linking the abducens nucleus in the pons to the

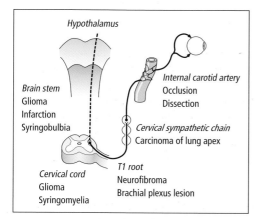

Figure 4.8 Causes of Horner's syndrome – classified according to the site of the lesion along the sympathetic pathway from the hypothalamus to the eye.

contralateral medial rectus part of the oculomotor nucleus in the midbrain. A lesion in this pathway results in successful abduction on attempted lateral gaze but failure of adduction of the other eye. There is also nystagmus, greater in the abducting eye. This combination, known as an internuclear ophthalmoplegia, is commonly encountered in multiple sclerosis (Chapter 16). Lesions of the medial longitudinal fasciculus may also produce **skew deviation**, in which one eye is elevated relative to the other in all gaze positions.

Conjugate gaze palsy

Complete or partial failure of both eyes to move in a particular direction (without diplopia, as the eyes remain aligned relative to each other) arises with **supranuclear** lesions of the pathways controlling eye movements, i.e. above the III, IV and VI nuclei. Such lesions may be compressive or acutely destructive, e.g. caused by infarction or haemorrhage. But a **supranuclear gaze palsy** may also be chronic and progressive in extrapyramidal neurodegenerative disease (Chapter 12). If, in the presence of a gaze palsy, eye movements are full on oculocephalic testing, the problem must be supranuclear.

Massive destructive lesions of the brainstem or cerebral hemisphere, sufficient to disturb consciousness as well as interfere with eye movement pathways, may result in **conjugate deviation** of the eyes (Fig. 4.9). The control centre for horizontal gaze is located in the pons (with higher centres in the cerebral hemispheres); that for vertical gaze is less well understood but involves structures in the superior midbrain.

Complex eye movement disorders

If the clinical findings do not fit neatly into one of the above categories, the patient may have a combination of nerve palsies (e.g., III, IV and VI palsies of one eye caused by a lesion in the cavernous sinus or superior orbital fissure – Chapter 13) or a bizarre brainstem lesion. But it is important also to think of more treatable conditions – Could the patient have **myasthenia gravis** (Chapter 17) or **dysthyroid eye disease** (Chapter 19)?

Testing diplopia

In many patients with binocular diplopia, the cause is obvious on testing eye movements when weakness of particular muscles becomes apparent. Sometimes, however, the defect is more subtle and the eye movements seem normal on pursuit testing, yet the patient still complains of diplopia. In such circumstances, it is first necessary to determine the direction where diplopia is maximal and how the two images are separated (horizontally, vertically or obliquely). Each eye is then covered in turn, and the image which disappears noted. As a general rule, the **false image** (from the affected eye) is always the outermost. Thus, for example, applying this **cover test** to a patient with a mild right lateral rectus palsy, diplopia is maximal on right gaze, with horizontal separation of the images. Covering the right eye, the outermost (further) image disappears, whereas covering the left eye, the nearer is lost.

V: Trigeminal nerve

Anatomy and examination

The trigeminal nerve is responsible for facial sensation (Fig. 4.10) and also innervates the masticatory muscles. Clinical examination of its motor function involves palpation of the bulk of the masseter and temporalis muscles, with the jaw tightly closed. The action of the pterygoid muscles can be assessed by asking the patient to open the jaw. With unilateral weakness, the jaw deviates towards the affected side because of the unopposed action of the normal muscle.

Sensory testing should include pinprick and light touch in each of the three divisions of the nerve (Fig. 4.10).

Peripheral trigeminal lesions produce sensory loss which follows these anatomical divisions. Central lesions, however, may involve the outer parts of the face, sparing the nose and mouth, in a 'balaclava helmet' distribution. This is because such lesions, if progressing upwards from the neck (e.g., syringobulbia, Chapter 15), may spare the uppermost part of the spinal nucleus of the trigeminal nerve, which serves the central part of the face.

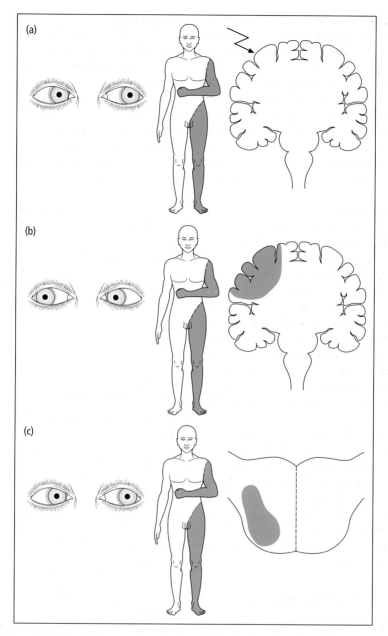

Figure 4.9 Conjugate deviation of the eyes. The direction of deviation is particularly useful in ascertaining the site of the lesion in hemiparetic patients with disturbed consciousness. (a) Partial epilepsy originating in one frontal lobe – eyes deviate towards affected limbs and away from the hemisphere containing the epileptic focus. (b) Destructive lesion of one frontal lobe – eyes deviate away from the hemiparetic side, due to the unopposed action of the higher centre for control of eye movement (frontal eye field) in the unaffected hemisphere. (c) Destructive unilateral brainstem (pontine) lesion – eyes deviate towards hemiparetic side. The lesion is above the pyramidal decussation, hence affecting the contralateral limbs. However, it is below the decussation of fibres from the frontal eye fields to the pons controlling horizontal eye movements. The unopposed action of the pontine gaze centre on the unaffected side of the brainstem deviates the eyes ipsilaterally.

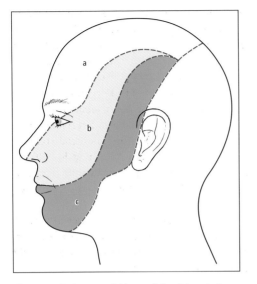

Figure 4.10 Sensory divisions of the trigeminal nerve: (a) ophthalmic, (b) maxillary, (c) mandibular. Note the trigeminal nerve is also responsible for innervation of non-cutaneous structures – the eye, particularly the cornea, the frontal and maxillary air sinuses, the nasal and oral cavities, including jaws, teeth and anterior two-thirds of tongue, and the temporomandibular joint and anterior wall of the external auditory meatus.

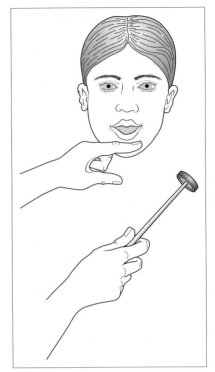

Figure 4.11 The jaw jerk.

The **corneal response** is tested by gently touching the edge of the cornea with a wisp of cotton wool and observing reflex blinking. The afferent arm of this reflex is conveyed by the trigeminal nerve (predominantly the ophthalmic division), but the efferent pathway is via the facial nerve to orbicularis oculi, the muscle responsible for eye closure. If there is ipsilateral facial weakness, intact corneal sensation may still be demonstrated by observing the consensual blink of the opposite eye.

The **jaw jerk** (Fig. 4.11) should also be assessed. In normal individuals it may be absent or just present, but it is pathologically brisk when there is bilateral upper motor neurone damage, affecting the lower cranial nerves (**pseudobulbar palsy** – see below).

Disorders

Trigeminal neuralgia

This is discussed in Chapter 9.

Trigeminal neuropathy

This, as evidenced by facial sensory loss, may occur in isolation. Alternatively, if unilateral, it may present in association with ipsilateral hearing loss, indicating a lesion at the cerebellopontine angle, e.g. an acoustic neuroma (Chapter 13). If bilateral, trigeminal sensory loss may form part of a more generalized sensory polyneuropathy (Chapter 17).

VII: Facial nerve

Anatomy and examination

In addition to supplying the muscles of facial expression, branches of the facial nerve serve other functions (Fig. 4.12). The involvement or sparing of these aspects can help localize the site of a lesion along the nerve.

The motor function of the nerve may be assessed first with the face at rest, where there may be

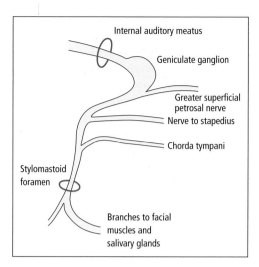

Figure 4.12 Facial nerve anatomy and function. Lesions in the region of the stylomastoid foramen produce facial paralysis alone. Proximal to the chorda tympani, a lesion will also affect taste sensation on the anterior two-thirds of the tongue. More proximal lesions may affect the nerve to stapedius (the patient complaining of heightened perception of sound – hyperacusis) and the greater superficial petrosal nerve (with ipsilateral loss of lacrimation).

obvious asymmetry, then by asking the patient in turn to raise the eyebrows, close the eyes tight, purse the lips, inflate the cheeks, grin, whistle and finally jut out the chin (to examine the contraction of platysma). With severe weakness of eye closure, patients may have difficulty protecting the cornea. Such patients can be seen to roll the eye upwards under the eyelid when asked to close the eyes, in an apparently automatic attempt to cover the cornea (**Bell's phenomenon** – a movement which occurs to a degree in everyone).

Weakness of the muscles of facial expression may be unilateral or bilateral. If unilateral, a useful distinction may be made between lower and upper motor neurone patterns of weakness. Lower motor neurone weakness, caused by damage to the facial nucleus in the brainstem or to the nerve itself, the 'final common path', involves all the muscles of facial expression. However, with upper motor neurone lesions, where the lesion lies between the contralateral cerebral cortex and the pons, the muscles of the upper part of the face (particularly frontalis,

responsible for raising the eyebrow and corrugating the forehead) may be spared. This is because the lower motor neurones to this part of the face are bilaterally innervated by corticopontine fibres. Thus, even if the neurones from the contralateral cortex are damaged, the ipsilateral innervation will still function. Furthermore, patients with upper motor neurone facial weakness can respond with normal facial movement in emotional contexts, e.g. laughter, even if the same muscles will not move to command. This is because the emotional and volitional upper motor neurone pathways are separate.

The sense of taste is assessed by carefully applying solutions representing the four basic gustatory modalities (sweet, salt, bitter and acid) to the anterior part of the tongue.

Disorders

Bell's palsy

This is an idiopathic unilateral lower motor neurone facial paralysis. It has been attributed to a viral or postviral phenomenon, with some evidence specifically for involvement of herpes simplex virus. The onset is rapid, within hours or at most days, and there may be associated pain in or behind the ear. Some physicians recommend corticosteroid and antiviral treatment if started during the first 48 hours of the illness. But even without this manoeuvre, 85–90% of patients recover completely, within weeks or months. Of the remainder, many have a satisfactory partial improvement. Only a very small minority are left with facial deformity. During the acute phase, a major priority is to protect the cornea, using artificial tears and/or taping the eyelid down. Patients with severe permanent lower motor neurone facial weakness may require the lateral parts of the upper and lower eyelid to be sutured together (**lateral tarsorrhaphy**) to protect the cornea.

Other causes of unilateral lower motor neurone facial paralysis are listed in Table 4.3. Upper motor neurone weakness is usually due to a pathological process in the contralateral cerebral hemisphere (e.g., infarction, tumour), and there may be

Table 4.3 Causes of lower motor neurone facial paralysis.

Brainstem Tumour, infarct, demyelination
Cerebellopontine angle Tumour (acoustic neuroma)
Petrous bone Middle ear infection Bell's palsy Herpes zoster
Face Parotid tumour and surgery Trauma
Other causes include meningeal infiltration or inflammation (malignant disease, sarcoid)

associated weakness of the limbs on the same side as the facial weakness. Bilateral facial weakness may be due to primary muscle disease (e.g., muscular dystrophies, Chapter 17) or disease at the neuromuscular junction (myasthenia gravis, Chapter 17). Indeed, the combination of a complex eye movement disorder with bilateral weakness of orbicularis oculi is almost pathognomonic of myasthenia. Lesions of both facial nerves may be acute (e.g., Guillain–Barré syndrome, Chapter 20). More chronic bilateral lesions suggest damage to the nerves in the basal meninges, e.g., as a result of malignant infiltration or sarcoidosis.

Hemifacial spasm

This is characterized by unilateral shock-like contractions of the facial muscles, typically occurring in elderly women. Treatment of this condition has been revolutionized by the use of botulinum toxin (Chapter 12).

VIII: Vestibulocochlear nerve

Hearing

Bedside tests of hearing include the patient's ability to detect a watch ticking close to the ear or repeat numbers whispered at a distance of approx-

imately 1 m from the ear, with the contralateral external auditory meatus blocked.

A 512-Hz tuning fork may be used to distinguish between **conductive** (external and middle ear) and **sensorineural** (inner ear, i.e. cochlea, and VIII nerve) hearing loss. In **Rinne's test**, air conduction (AC), with the vibrating fork placed in front of the ear, is compared with bone conduction (BC), with the base of the fork against the mastoid process. Normally, AC > BC, but with conductive hearing loss, BC > AC. With sensorineural loss, AC > BC, but both are reduced compared with the normal ear. In **Weber's test**, the base of the vibrating fork is placed on the centre of the forehead. Normally, sound is heard in the middle. With sensorineural hearing loss, sound is lateralized towards the normal side, but with conductive loss, sound lateralizes towards the affected side.

Balance

Anatomy

The vestibular division of the VIII nerve conveys sensory information from the vestibular apparatus of the inner ear (the labyrinth, comprising the three semicircular canals, utricle and saccule) to the vestibular nuclei of the brainstem and to the cerebellum. The vestibular nuclei have complex connections with the cerebellum and with the III, IV and VI nuclei, as well as projections to the cerebral cortex. Normal balance depends on the integrity of this system, along with inputs from the eyes and from sensory receptors in the neck, trunk and limbs.

Symptoms

Vertigo is a false perception of movement, either of the patient or of their surroundings, as a result of an imbalance of the vestibular inputs. Some patients experience severe vertigo, with the world appearing to rotate around them, and associated nausea, vomiting and loss of balance. Milder symptoms may be described as the patients' feeling as if they are on a boat. 'Dizziness' is a very common presenting symptom – care must be taken to establish whether the patient is really complaining of vertigo, or whether there is some other intended meaning, e.g. unsteadiness of gait or pre-syncope.

The presence of associated symptoms may help localize lesions in the vestibular pathways. Thus, vertigo alone or in combination with cochlear symptoms (hearing loss, tinnitus) suggests a peripheral vestibular (labyrinthine or VIII nerve) disturbance. The coexistence of vertigo and diplopia indicates central (brainstem) disease, whereas diplopia without vertigo is more consistent with an efferent lesion of the III, IV and/or VI nerves, or the muscles they innervate.

Examination

Nystagmus may be found in patients with vertigo. With labyrinthine disease, nystagmus is horizontal or rotatory and beats away from the side of the lesion (as opposed to cerebellar disease, where it beats towards the side of the lesion). The mechanism underlying labyrinthine nystagmus is that an imbalance between the two inner ears will cause the eyes to deviate towards the side of the lesion, with fast corrective saccades towards the opposite side, counterbalancing this slow component.

Vestibular nystagmus is worsened by turning the head in the direction of the fast phase. Indeed, sudden head movement is a means of provoking nystagmus in patients with peripheral vestibular lesions (as in the **Hallpike manoeuvre**, see below). **Caloric testing** or rotation in a specially designed chair is a means of provoking vestibular nystagmus in normal individuals. In a conscious patient, the caloric test involves instilling cold (30°C) or, less commonly, warm (44°C) water into each external auditory meatus. Nystagmus induced by the cold water normally persists for approximately 2 minutes. Damage to the vestibular apparatus may reduce the response in one direction (**canal paresis**) but sometimes, when spontaneous nystagmus is present, it is increased in one direction by caloric testing (**directional preponderance**).

Examination of a vertiginous patient should also include hearing tests and the detection of other cranial nerve lesions. In **Romberg's test**

Table 4.4 Causes of dizziness.

General medical
Cardiovascular (postural hypotension, dysrhythmias)
Metabolic (hypoglycaemia, hyperventilation)
Anaemia, polycythaemia
Neurological
Syncope
Vascular disease
Tumour, particularly acoustic neuroma
Cerebellar/brainstem disorders (e.g., multiple sclerosis)
Migraine
Epilepsy
Otological
Ototoxic drugs, particularly aminoglycosides
Post-traumatic
Other inner ear disorders (see text)
Secondary to middle ear disease
In elderly patients, more than one pathology may contribute to dizziness. Minor dysfunction of two or more of the sensory inputs responsible for normal balance (vestibular, visual, proprioceptive), e.g. due to cataracts, arthritis, labyrinthine damage, in combination with cerebrovascular disease, may result in the 'multisensory dizziness syndrome'
Sedative drugs may also make patients dizzy (antidepressants, anti-epilepsy drugs, benzodiazepines, alcohol)

(Chapter 5), patients with acute labyrinthine lesions will tend to fall towards the affected side. Gait may be mildly unsteady. General examination is also important, in particular looking for postural hypotension (Chapter 7).

Disorders

Causes of dizziness, both vertiginous and non-vertiginous, are listed in Table 4.4. Some of the more common conditions are considered in more detail below.

Acute labyrinthitis

This is assumed to be a viral or postviral condition in which the patient typically wakes with severe vertigo, exacerbated by head movement, and often associated with nausea and vomiting. The acute phase may last several days, during which nystagmus may be evident. Later, there is gradual improvement but mild symptoms, provoked by head movement, may persist for months. During the recovery phase, nystagmus disappears but a unilateral canal paresis may be detected. Treatment with a **vestibular sedative**, e.g. cinnarizine, may be beneficial when the symptoms are severe.

Benign paroxysmal positional vertigo (BPPV)

This condition, also known as benign positioning vertigo, arises from the presence of debris (otoconia) in the posterior semicircular canal, as a result of degeneration of the balance sensory organs of the utricle. Such damage may be idiopathic or may follow labyrinthitis or head injury ('labyrinthine concussion'). When the head moves, turbulent flow within the endolymph of the semicircular canal, because of the otoconial debris, produces transient recurrent positional vertigo.

BPPV is associated with characteristic abnormalities of the **Hallpike manoeuvre**. This involves gently but rapidly lowering the patient backwards from a sitting position so that their head hangs over the end of the bed, first turned to the right, then repeated turned to the left. In BPPV, nystagmus and vertigo develop after a delay of several seconds, last up to 1 minute, and fatigue with repeat testing. By contrast, central (brainstem) vestibular lesions are characterized by nystagmus without vertigo on the Hallpike manoeuvre, and there is no latent period and no fatigability on repeat testing.

BPPV is typically provoked by particular head postures, e.g. lying with the head turned to one side, or neck extension. The patient may learn to avoid these positions and may benefit from vestibular sedatives. More recently, manoeuvres have been developed to disperse the otoconial debris (Epley manoeuvre).

Ménière's disease

This condition is due to increased pressure in the membranous labyrinth. It is characterized by attacks of severe vertigo, typically occurring in clusters (several episodes in a few weeks) separated by periods of remission. The vertigo is associated with tinnitus and hearing loss, which persists between attacks and may gradually worsen. Vestibular sedatives may be beneficial during acute episodes.

Vertebrobasilar ischaemia

This is commonly associated with vertigo, but can only be invoked with certainty as the cause of this symptom if other features of posterior circulation ischaemia (Chapter 11) are present.

Chronic persistent vertigo

This warrants detailed neuro-otological assessment. Most patients, however, still have a peripheral vestibular disorder. Treatment consists of vestibular rehabilitation exercises, taught by a physiotherapist.

IX and X: Glossopharyngeal and vagus nerves

Though the glossopharyngeal nerve has many functions, the only aspect that is routinely tested clinically is common sensation on the posterior pharyngeal wall and the posterior third of the tongue. Anything more than a gentle stimulus to these regions with an orange stick will produce a **gag reflex** – contraction of the pharynx, retraction of the tongue and elevation of the palate.

The efferent limb of the gag reflex is conveyed via the vagus nerve. This nerve also has multiple functions, and several aspects other than the motor component of the gag reflex are amenable to clinical examination:

- Swallowing – Can the patient drink a glass of water without nasal regurgitation of liquid (suggesting **palatal incompetence**) or coughing (because of spillage of fluid into the trachea)?
- Palatal movement – elevation during phonation (say 'ah') should be observed: with unilateral weakness, the palate and uvula are pulled towards the normal side.
- Speech – there may be impaired articulation (**dysarthria** – see below); the voice may be hoarse or husky.
- Coughing – typically 'bovine', i.e. without its usual explosive quality in vagal lesions. Unilateral or bilateral vocal cord paralysis in vagus lesions

will also render the patient unable to utter high-pitched noises ('eeee') or to sing.

XI: Accessory nerve

This nerve supplies the sternomastoid and trapezius muscles. Wasting of one or both sternomastoids is usually obvious. Power of these muscles is assessed by asking the patient to turn the head against resistance. The left sternomastoid turns the head to the right and vice versa. Combined action of the sternomastoids results in neck flexion. Trapezius is assessed by asking the patient to shrug the shoulders against resistance.

XII: Hypoglossal nerve

This nerve supplies the tongue muscles. A lower motor neurone lesion results in unilateral or bilateral wasting and fasciculation (Chapter 5), best observed with the tongue at rest in the floor of the mouth. On protrusion, unilateral weakness leads to deviation of the tongue towards the affected side. Side-to-side movements of the tongue may be impaired and slow with bilateral wasting and weakness, but this is more commonly a sign of bilateral upper motor neurone (corticobulbar) damage.

Dysarthria

Articulation of speech must be distinguished from higher-order language function and its disorders – dysphasia (Chapter 3). Normal articulation depends on coordination of the larynx, pharynx, tongue, lips and respiration by means of corticobulbar, bulbar, cerebellar and extrapyramidal pathways.

In addition to assessing the patient's conversational speech, certain test phrases should be repeated, e.g. 'baby hippopotamus', 'West Register Street' and 'British Constitution'.

Lesions of specific parts of the controlling neural pathways may produce characteristic speech abnormalities:

- palatal paralysis – 'nasal' speech quality;

Table 4.5 Bulbar and pseudobulbar palsy.

Bulbar	Pseudobulbar
Causes	
Brainstem vascular disease	Bihemispheric vascular disease
Motor neurone disease	Motor neurone disease
Syringobulbia	Multiple sclerosis
Tumour	Tumour
Brainstem encephalitis (e.g., polio)	Extrapyramidal disease
Multiple cranial nerve palsies (e.g., Guillain–Barré syndrome)	
Skull base or meningeal infiltration	
Myasthenia gravis	
Some muscular dystrophies	
Polymyositis	
Features	
Nasal speech	Slow, monotonous speech, sometimes explosive
Absent jaw jerk	Brisk jaw jerk
Palatal weakness, nasal regurgitation of food	Dysphagia
Reduced or absent gag reflex	Brisk gag reflex
Wasted, fasciculating tongue	Shrunken, immobile tongue
	Emotional lability with spontaneous laughing and crying
	Associated upper motor neurone signs in limbs

- cerebellar lesions – slurred speech, with an irregular staccato or scanning quality;
- extrapyramidal disease – monotonous, soft speech;
- bilateral corticobulbar damage – slow, grunting, 'spastic' speech.

Bulbar and pseudobulbar palsy

Lesions of cranial nerves IX–XII at nuclear (brainstem), nerve or muscle level (bulbar palsy) differ from bilateral upper motor neurone (corticobulbar) lesions to the lower brainstem (pseudobulbar palsy), in both clinical features and causes, as summarized in Table 4.5. In motor neurone disease, bulbar and pseudobulbar features may coexist (Chapter 18).

Key points

- The diagnosis of lesions in the visual pathways relies on detailed examination of all the upper cranial nerves
- Clinical assessment of the optic nerve comprises several components: visual acuity, fields, colour vision, fundoscopy, pupillary responses (afferent part)
- Examining pursuit eye movements is a rapid screening test for ocular motility disorders
- In an unconscious patient, lesion localization may be aided by examination of eye movements (e.g., vestibulo-ocular reflex, conjugate deviation) and pupils
- Lesions of the lower cranial nerves, affecting swallowing and articulation of speech (hence dysarthria), may be classified as bulbar (lower motor neurone) or pseudobulbar (upper motor neurone)

Chapter 5

Motor function

The production of complex yet smoothly coordinated movement is dependent on the integrity of much of the nervous system:

- higher centres (Chapter 3),
- upper motor neurone (UMN),
- lower motor neurone (LMN),
- neuromuscular junction (Chapter 17),
- muscle (Chapter 17);

with important input from:

- basal ganglia–extrapyramidal pathways (Chapter 12),
- cerebellum;

and 'feedback' via sensory pathways, particularly conveying information about joint position (Chapter 6).

UMN and LMN

There are many motor pathways descending from the cerebral cortex and brainstem. However, for the purpose of classifying disorders of voluntary movement, the UMN may be considered synonymous with neurones whose cell bodies are in the **motor cortex** and whose axons run in the **corticospinal (pyramidal) tracts** to synapse with **anterior horn cells** (Fig. 5.1). These neurones may be considered the anatomical substrate for the

Lecture Notes: Neurology, 9th edition. By Lionel Ginsberg. Published 2010 by Blackwell Publishing.

initiation of willed movements, particularly fine or complex manipulations.

The LMN is the 'final common path' of the motor system, with axons extending from the anterior horn cells of the spinal cord to the voluntary muscles. One anterior horn cell supplies many muscle fibres – forming a **motor unit**.

Examination of the motor system

Motor function in the limbs should be examined clinically in the order given in Table 5.1.

Patterns of abnormality of these seven aspects, along with information from observing the patient's **gait** and **stance**, and from examining for neck and trunk weakness, will generally help localize a lesion within the motor system.

Wasting

Loss of muscle bulk is typically less prominent in primary muscle disease (**myopathy**) than in conditions where muscles have been denervated (**neurogenic wasting**) as a result of LMN lesions. Wasting is not a feature of UMN lesions, though prolonged disuse may produce some atrophy.

The distribution of neurogenic wasting will depend on which LMNs have been damaged, and whether the damage has been at anterior horn cell level, or distally at the spinal roots or individual peripheral nerves. Certain patterns of wasting

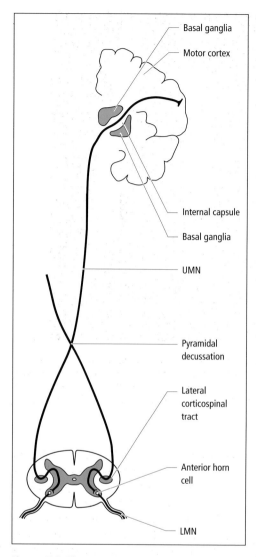

Figure 5.1 Diagrammatic representation of the corticospinal tract. The UMN descends from the motor cortex through the internal capsule. Most fibres decussate in the medulla to form the lateral corticospinal tracts in the spinal cord, then synapse with LMNs (usually indirectly via an interneurone – not shown) at anterior horn cell level.

Labels in figure: Basal ganglia; Motor cortex; Internal capsule; Basal ganglia; UMN; Pyramidal decussation; Lateral corticospinal tract; Anterior horn cell; LMN

Table 5.1 Order of examination of the motor system.

Wasting
Involuntary movements
Tone
Posture
Power
Coordination
Reflexes

set of options. This is shown in Fig. 5.3, where the common clinical situation of a patient presenting with wasting of the intrinsic muscles of one hand is considered.

Involuntary movements

Fasciculations are brief, irregular twitching movements visible through the skin and occurring within a muscle belly. They are insufficiently powerful to achieve movement around the joint served by the muscle, except sometimes in the hand. They indicate an LMN lesion, generally proximal and severe, especially at anterior horn cell level. Some benign fasciculations, particularly in the calf muscles, are of no pathological significance.

Other involuntary movements are of greater amplitude and often signify disease of the extrapyramidal system (Chapter 12).

Tone

Muscle tone may be defined clinically as the resistance detected by the examiner on passive movement of a patient's joints, hence **passive stretch** of the muscles. Some resistance is observed in normal individuals, but it may be increased or decreased by disease (**hyper-** and **hypotonia**, respectively).

The phenomenon of muscle tone and many other physical signs of motor function depend on the integrity of the **stretch reflex** shown in idealized form in Fig. 5.4. Passive stretch of a muscle induces afferent impulses to the spinal cord, which in turn activate the motor neurone, leading to reflex contraction. As the clinical correlate of this

occur relatively commonly and these areas should be inspected routinely (Fig. 5.2).

Inspection alone is often sufficient to achieve some anatomical localization; as with other areas of neurology, the examiner should look logically for a feature that discriminates between a limited

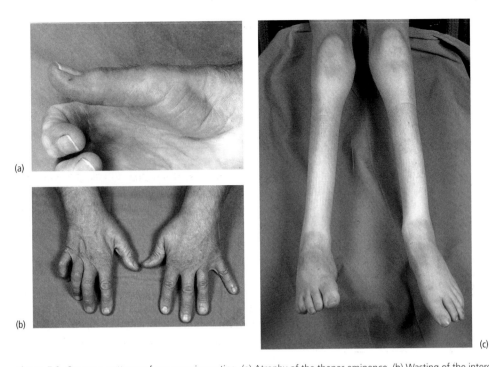

(a)

(b)

(c)

Figure 5.2 Common patterns of neurogenic wasting. (a) Atrophy of the thenar eminence. (b) Wasting of the interossei; the affected right hand (which is also clawed) may be compared with the left, which is normal. (c) Severe distal lower limb wasting. With milder degrees of wasting of tibialis anterior, an early sign is loss of the smooth contour of the shin, the anterior border of the tibia becoming more prominent. Upper and lower limbs should also be inspected for more proximal wasting (particularly the periscapular and thigh muscles).

response is normal muscle tone, it follows that interruption of the reflex arc by disease, for example by LMN damage, will lead to a reduction in tone or hypotonia – the muscle will become **flaccid**.

Disease affecting the UMN in turn produces hypertonia or **spasticity**. The reason for this is not so much damage to the excitatory UMN itself but rather dysfunction of polysynaptic pathways descending in parallel with it, which exert an in-

hibitory effect on the LMN and hence on the reflex arc. Loss of **supraspinal inhibition** unmasks the stretch reflex in a more primitive or 'undamped' form, and tone is thereby increased.

The characteristic quality of hypertonia caused by UMN damage is that there is marked resistance to passive muscle stretch through part of the range of movement of a joint, but at a certain point the resistance suddenly 'gives' (**clasp-knife**

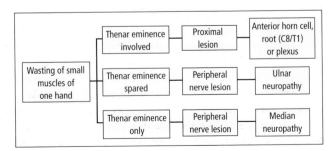

Figure 5.3 Algorithm for analysing the causes of wasting of the intrinsic muscles of one hand.

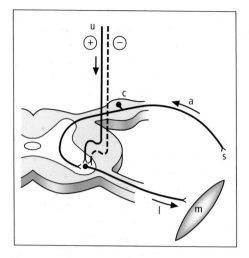

Figure 5.4 The stretch reflex. s, stretch receptor; a, afferent (sensory) neurone; c, cell body of sensory neurone in dorsal root ganglion; l, LMN originating at anterior horn cell of spinal cord; m, muscle; u, UMN; arrows indicate direction of impulse traffic; +, excitatory impulse in UMN; −, inhibitory impulse in parallel descending inhibitory pathways. Not all the components of the reflex are shown. The descending inhibitory pathways mainly act on the gamma efferents (not shown) which modulate the sensitivity of the stretch receptors.

phenomenon). In some patients with subtle UMN lesions, the only feature of such a lesion in the upper limbs may be a miniature version of the clasp-knife effect, elicited by supinating and pronating the forearm (**supinator catch**).

Other forms of increased tone, caused by extrapyramidal disease, are described in Chapter 12.

Posture

Another sign of mild upper limb UMN damage may be observed with the patient's arms outstretched, palms facing upwards and eyes shut. An affected limb will first pronate then drift downwards (**pronator** or **pyramidal drift** sign).

Disease of other parts of the nervous system may also be identified by asking the patient to perform this simple manoeuvre. For example, a patient with loss of joint position sense in the hands may show irregular involuntary movements of the fingers when the arm is outstretched and the eyes

are shut ('**pseudoathetosis**'), because of loss of all avenues of sensory input relating to maintenance of this posture (**deafferentation**).

Postural abnormalities as a result of extrapyramidal disease are again described in Chapter 12.

Power

Power is assessed clinically by grading the patient's ability to contract a muscle voluntarily against gravity and against resistance provided by the examiner. The **Medical Research Council scale** is used most commonly in the UK:

0 no contraction,
1 flicker or trace of contraction,
2 active movement, with gravity eliminated,
3 active movement against gravity,
4 active movement against gravity and resistance,
5 normal power.

This scale is at best semiquantitative, particularly as much muscle weakness (**paresis**) in clinical neurology falls within the 3–5 range, where it is often necessary to make further subjective subdivisions, i.e. 4−, 4 and 4+, denoting severe, moderate and mild weakness respectively.

For most 'screening' examinations, it is sufficient to test an agonist–antagonist muscle pair at each of the major joints (Fig. 5.5). Right- and left-sided limbs should be compared at each joint because weakness is often asymmetrical and patients may therefore act as their own 'controls'.

Although it is possible to assess power exhaustively in many other limb muscles, selection is required. This is generally governed by information already available from the history, or from other parts of the examination, whereby a particular pattern of focal weakness may have suggested itself. Anatomical localization is then achieved once again by discriminating between very few options as shown for the very common clinical problems of wrist and foot drop (Fig. 5.6). Likewise, the history may have pointed to a lesion of an individual cervical spinal segment (neck pain radiating down one arm), again a very common clinical situation (Chapter 15). In this case, the aim is to detect a pattern of weakness corresponding to the muscles innervated by a single segmental nerve, its **myotome** (Table 5.2). More diffuse processes affecting many nerves or muscles simultaneously, e.g. metabolic or inflammatory, may produce more generalized weakness but specific patterns remain discernible. Thus, primary muscle disease is typically associated with proximal weakness whereas a motor polyneuropathy usually produces distal weakness.

UMN lesions are also associated with characteristic patterns of weakness. Unlike LMN lesions, these relate more to voluntary movements than to individual muscles, the UMN being at a higher level of organization in the nervous system. A time-honoured term referring to UMN weakness in the limbs is the '**pyramidal distribution**' of weakness. By this is meant greater weakness of extensors than flexors in the upper limbs and of flexors than extensors in the lower limbs. Formal objective measurement of muscle power in UMN lesions using a strain gauge (**myometry**) has cast doubt on this pattern. However, the description remains of clinical value, particularly as it corresponds to abnormalities of posture seen in patients with advanced UMN lesions. Thus, a patient who is **hemiparetic** after a vascular event in one cerebral hemisphere will typically have a flexed arm and extended leg on the opposite side of the body from the brain lesion.

Coordination

Lack of coordination, or **ataxia**, is often considered synonymous with cerebellar disease. But, as previously stated, coordinated movement requires the normal action of all the components of the motor system and of parts of the sensory system, particularly joint position sense. Thus, loss of position sense may lead to a **sensory ataxia**. In the hand, this may have as damaging an effect on *useful* movement as severe muscle weakness.

Formal tests of coordination in the limbs may, however, provide localizing information on cerebellar disease, the lesion generally being in the cerebellar hemisphere on the same side as the abnormal sign.

In the upper limb, the cardinal test of coordination is the **finger–nose–finger test**, where the patient moves his or her index finger backwards and forwards from his or her nose to the examiner's finger. Cerebellar disease leads to inaccuracy in this test (**past-pointing**) because of inability to judge distances (**dysmetria**). As the finger approaches the target, it may oscillate increasingly wildly (**intention tremor**). An alternative test is to ask the patient to perform **rapid alternating movements** (e.g., by tapping the dorsum of one hand with the palmar and then the dorsal aspect of the fingers of the opposite hand repeatedly), which may be jerky and inaccurate in cerebellar disease (**dysdiadochokinesis**). Dysmetria may also be assessed by gently tapping the patient's outstretched hand. Rather than immediately returning to the initial position, the patient's arm may overshoot and oscillate a few times (**cerebellar rebound**).

In the lower limbs, ataxia may be detected in the **heel–knee–shin test**, the patient being asked to place one heel on the opposite knee then slide it accurately down the shin. These tests of limb ataxia provide only a partial picture of cerebellar function. Much may also be learnt from assessment of muscle tone, which may be reduced in cerebellar disease, from the reflexes (see below) and from examining:

- gait (see below),
- speech (Chapter 4),
- eye movements (Chapter 4).

Reflexes

Tendon reflexes

These are a direct method of testing the immediate action of the stretch reflex clinically. Striking the tendon of a muscle with a patellar hammer will stretch the muscle passively and induce reflex contraction. As with muscle tone, tendon reflexes may be heightened or diminished by disease.

Interruption of the reflex arc, for example by LMN damage, will render the reflex depressed or absent. Sometimes a reflex that initially appears

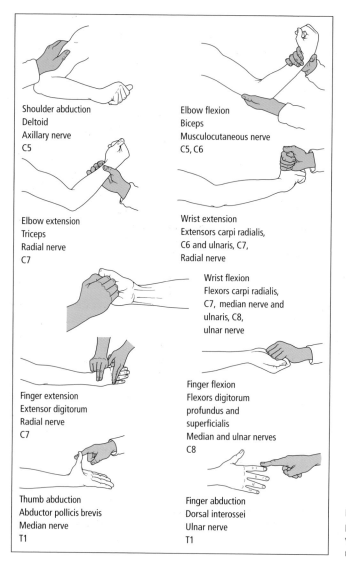

Shoulder abduction
Deltoid
Axillary nerve
C5

Elbow flexion
Biceps
Musculocutaneous nerve
C5, C6

Elbow extension
Triceps
Radial nerve
C7

Wrist extension
Extensors carpi radialis,
C6 and ulnaris, C7,
Radial nerve

Wrist flexion
Flexors carpi radialis,
C7, median nerve and
ulnaris, C8,
ulnar nerve

Finger extension
Extensor digitorum
Radial nerve
C7

Finger flexion
Flexors digitorum
profundus and
superficialis
Median and ulnar nerves
C8

Thumb abduction
Abductor pollicis brevis
Median nerve
T1

Finger abduction
Dorsal interossei
Ulnar nerve
T1

Figure 5.5 Clinical testing of muscle power. For each movement, the relevant muscle, peripheral nerve and main root value are given.

absent may be obtained by asking the patient to clench his or her teeth (for upper limb reflexes) or to interlock the fingers of the right hand with those of the left then try to pull the hands apart (for lower limb reflexes, **Jendrassik's manoeuvre**), at the same time as the examiner strikes the tendon. This phenomenon of **reinforcement** is due to such manoeuvres increasing the sensitivity of stretch receptors throughout the body.

UMN lesions may produce brisk tendon reflexes as a result of loss of supraspinal inhibition. **Clonus** is a physical sign most often elicited at the ankle where sudden but maintained dorsiflexion by the examiner (with the patient's knee also partially flexed) produces rhythmical repetitive alternating plantar flexion and dorsiflexion. This is also due to loss of supraspinal inhibition, the sharp muscle stretching, leading to oscillation within the circuit of the reflex arc. Clonus may be sustained or may

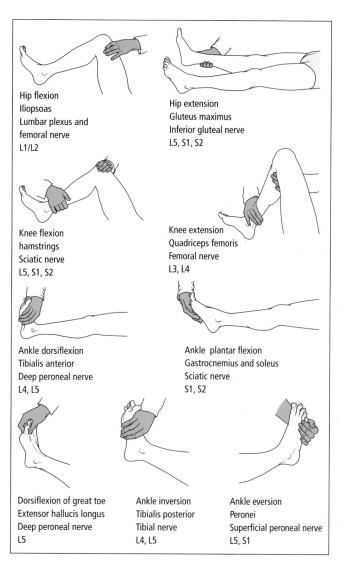

Hip flexion
Iliopsoas
Lumbar plexus and
femoral nerve
L1/L2

Hip extension
Gluteus maximus
Inferior gluteal nerve
L5, S1, S2

Knee flexion
hamstrings
Sciatic nerve
L5, S1, S2

Knee extension
Quadriceps femoris
Femoral nerve
L3, L4

Ankle dorsiflexion
Tibialis anterior
Deep peroneal nerve
L4, L5

Ankle plantar flexion
Gastrocnemius and soleus
Sciatic nerve
S1, S2

Dorsiflexion of great toe
Extensor hallucis longus
Deep peroneal nerve
L5

Ankle inversion
Tibialis posterior
Tibial nerve
L4, L5

Ankle eversion
Peronei
Superficial peroneal nerve
L5, S1

Figure 5.5 (*Continued*)

persist for only a few '**beats**'. It may be present in normal individuals, particularly if symmetrical in duration. It is of pathological significance if asymmetrical or if there is sustained symmetrical ankle clonus in the presence of other UMN signs. Clonus at sites other than the ankles (knees, fingers) is also generally pathological.

The grading of tendon reflexes is usually represented symbolically as follows:

+++ very brisk,
++ brisk,
+ present,
± with reinforcement,
0 absent,
CL clonus.

The main clinical usefulness of the tendon reflexes is in localizing lesions, especially of the

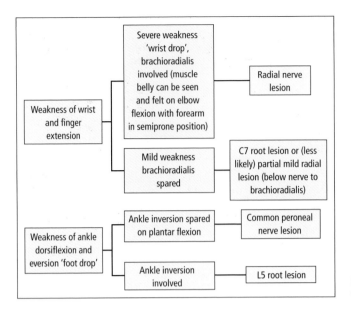

Figure 5.6 Algorithms for analysing the causes of wrist and foot drop.

spinal cord. This arises because the reflexes have **'root values'**, i.e. the relevant afferent and efferent nerves are located in particular spinal segments (Fig. 5.7). Thus, for example, a lesion of the spinal cord at C5/6 may abolish the biceps and the

Table 5.2 Segmental innervation of selected upper limb muscles.*

C5
Most shoulder movements, e.g. abduction
Biceps
C6
Brachioradialis
Extensor carpi radialis longus (extension and abduction at wrist)
C7
Triceps
Extensor carpi ulnaris (extension and adduction at wrist)
Finger extension
C8
Wrist flexion (and adduction)
Finger flexion
T1
Intrinsic muscles of hand

* Most of these muscles are innervated by fibres from more than one root, e.g. the 'root value' of brachioradialis is in fact C5/6 but C6 predominates.

supinator reflexes, because of LMN damage at that level, but all reflexes below (triceps downwards) will be brisk, because of UMN damage and hence loss of supraspinal inhibition of those segments – a **'reflex level'**.

Tendon reflexes may possess qualities indicative of disease processes other than those directly affecting the motor neurones, e.g. the slow-relaxing reflex of hypothyroidism and the pendular reflex of cerebellar disease.

Cutaneous reflexes

The cutaneous reflexes most often of value clinically are the **plantar** and **superficial abdominal responses**. These depend on afferent nerves concerned with pain sensation (**nociception**).

The normal response in adults to a stroke along the skin of the lateral border of the foot with an orange stick is plantar flexion of the toes ('downgoing' plantar response). In normal infants, there is a more primitive version of this flexor withdrawal reflex, with dorsiflexion of the great toe and abduction (**fanning**) of the other toes ('upgoing' plantar response). It is this version which reappears in adult life in the context of UMN damage (**positive Babinski reflex**).

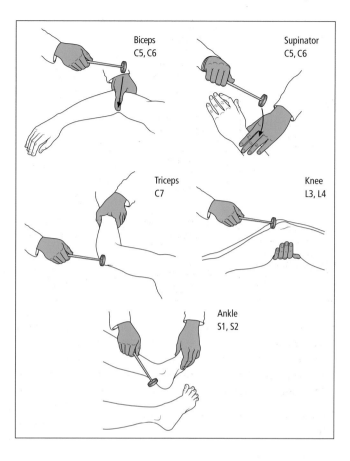

Figure 5.7 The tendon reflexes.

The superficial abdominal responses are elicited by a swift stroke with an orange stick horizontally across the skin of each abdominal quadrant. Normally there is reflex contraction of the underlying abdominal muscles, but this may be lost in UMN lesions (e.g., loss of the abdominal responses may be an early sign of multiple sclerosis).

The superficial abdominal responses may also be absent in obese patients, in those with abdominal scars and after repeated pregnancy.

Neck and trunk

Neck flexion is achieved by simultaneous contraction of both sternomastoid muscles,

Table 5.3 Neurological gait disorders.

Spastic paraparesis (UMN lesions, both legs)	Scissoring, 'wading through mud'
Spastic hemiparesis (UMN lesion, one side of body)	Leg is rigid and circumducts (describes a semicircle rotating at hip)
Bilateral foot drop (LMN lesions, both legs)	Steppage – legs lifted high to avoid scraping toe
Cerebellar lesion	Wide-based gait, staggering, unable to walk heel–toe
Parkinsonism	Stooping posture, rigid shuffling gait, 'festinant', no arm swing
Proximal myopathy	Waddling

innervated by the spinal accessory nerves (Chapter 4). Weakness of neck extension, such that the patient has to support his or her head with hand under chin, is relatively uncommon, but occurs in:

- myasthenia gravis (Chapter 17),
- polymyositis (Chapter 17),
- motor neurone disease (Chapter 18).

Truncal weakness, detected by asking the patient to rise unaided from a lying to a sitting position with arms folded, may occur as part of a more generalized proximal weakness, as seen in primary muscle disease.

Truncal ataxia is particularly associated with damage to cerebellar midline (**vermis**) structures. It may be so severe that the patient is unable to maintain a stable sitting posture unsupported.

Gait and stance

Certain gaits are associated with specific neurological disorders (Table 5.3).

Much may also be learnt from observing the patient standing unaided. A patient who falls when asked to stand 'to attention' with eyes shut is likely to have impaired joint position sense at the ankles (**Romberg's sign**).

Key points		
	LMN	**UMN**
Wasting	Present (neurogenic wasting)	Disuse atrophy only
Fasciculations	May be present	Absent
Tone	Normal or decreased (flaccidity)	Increased (spasticity)
Posture	–	Drift of outstretched arm (eyes shut)
Power	Focal weakness, e.g. distribution of individual nerves or roots	Movement-based Pyramidal distribution
Tendon reflexes	Depressed or absent	Brisk
Clonus	Absent	May be present
Plantar response	Downgoing or absent	Upgoing (positive Babinski)
Superficial abdominal responses	Present	May be absent
Gait	May be high-stepping	Spastic, scissoring, circumduction

Further reading

Note: Also relevant for Chapters 6, 15 and 17.

O'Brien MD (on behalf of the Guarantors of *Brain*). *Aids to the Examination of the Peripheral Nervous System*, 4th edn. WB Saunders, London, 2000.

(A guide to the motor and sensory examination of the peripheral nerves and nerve roots, all in a single portable volume).

Chapter 6

Sensation

The basic modalities of sensation that are tested as part of the routine clinical examination are:

- position sense,
- vibration sense,
- touch and pressure,
- pain and temperature (nociception).

Clinical neuroanatomy

There are two main neural pathways relaying sensory information from the peripheral receptors to the cerebral cortex, each consisting of three neurones.

Position and **vibration sense** are conveyed by a pathway involving the posterior columns of the spinal cord. Here, impulses from receptors travel via a primary sensory neurone to the cord, entering by a dorsal root. A central process of the same neurone ascends in the posterior columns to the brainstem. Only at this point does information cross to the opposite side of the nervous system, via a second neurone after synaptic transmission in the medulla. A third neurone projects from the thalamus to the cerebral cortex (parietal lobe).

Pain and **temperature** are conveyed by a pathway involving the spinothalamic tracts in the

cord. Here the primary sensory neurone again enters the cord via a dorsal root. But after a synapse in the cord itself, information ascends to the thalamus by the contralateral spinothalamic tract, the second sensory neurone having crossed over at, or within a few segments above, the level of entry of the primary neurone. The third neurone is again thalamocortical.

Touch and **pressure** sensation ascend the spinal cord by more than one route, both anterior and posterior.

Thus, the posterior columns largely convey **uncrossed** sensory information, whereas in the spinothalamic tracts, it is **crossed**. This difference in the level of the decussation in the major sensory pathways explains the distribution of sensory deficits seen in spinal cord disease (Chapter 15).

Practical points

Sensory symptoms

Patients may report negative symptoms as a result of damage to sensory pathways, e.g. numbness, inability to detect heat and cold. As elsewhere in neurology, there are also spontaneous positive symptoms, e.g. tingling, 'pins and needles' and other abnormal sensations (**paraesthesiae**). **Dysaesthesiae** are unpleasant distorted sensations arising from actual sensory stimuli. Chronic pain may also result from damage to sensory

Lecture Notes: Neurology, 9th edition. By Lionel Ginsberg. Published 2010 by Blackwell Publishing.

pathways, e.g. **thalamic pain**, experienced on the opposite side of the body to the site of the lesion in the thalamus.

Sensory signs

An overriding consideration when conducting the sensory examination of a patient is its **subjectivity**. It is therefore best performed after the motor examination, including the reflexes, has been completed. Because of this subjectivity, the examiner may easily be misled either by a patient's excessive desire to be helpful or, less frequently, by deliberate misinformation from a malingering patient. One must always be wary of sensory signs elicited in the absence of symptoms. The sensory examination is best conducted rapidly as this is less tiring for examiner and patient, and speed will reduce any opportunities for false information to be given.

Those modalities of sensation less likely to be prone to error from subjectivity are best tested first, as follows.

Position sense

This is assessed by determining a patient's ability to detect upward and downward passive movement of the fingers and toes with the eyes shut. An error rate greater than that expected on a chance basis should raise the suspicion of malingering. If distal position sense is impaired, more proximal joints should be tested. **Romberg's sign** (Chapter 5) is primarily a test of position sense at the ankles.

Vibration sense

This is tested with a 128-Hz tuning fork. The patient's ability to detect vibration when the base of the fork is placed on the sternum should first be confirmed. A similar sensation normally should then be appreciable at the extremities. If the patient cannot detect vibration at the fingers and toes, more proximal bony prominences should be tested, e.g. the malleoli at the ankles and the ulnar styloid at the wrist. Greater objectivity may be achieved by ensuring that the patient can distin-

guish between the application of a vibrating and non-vibrating fork with the eyes shut, and can determine the duration of the vibration.

Cutaneous sensation

This includes ability to detect:
- light touch using a cotton wool ball,
- painful stimuli using a pinprick,
- temperature using a metal cylinder filled with hot or cold water.

The limits of an area of sensory loss should be determined by moving the stimulus and asking the patient to report as soon as sensation returns to normal. Greater objectivity may be reached by determining whether the patient can distinguish between a pinprick and a more blunt stimulus, or between hot and cold, with the eyes shut. Similarly, a patient may be asked to close the eyes and report every time the light touch of a cotton wool ball is detected.

Patterns of sensory loss

Damage to an individual peripheral nerve may result in an area of cutaneous sensory loss corresponding to the entire extent of the skin supplied by that nerve (e.g., Fig. 6.1a). But if a toxic or metabolic insult has affected multiple peripheral nerves (polyneuropathy), the initial involvement of the longest nerves produces a characteristic 'glove-and-stocking' pattern of sensory loss in the extremities (Fig. 6.1b). Sensory nerve root damage may again lead to cutaneous sensory loss affecting the entire area of skin (**dermatome**) supplied by the root in question (Fig. 6.1c). The dermatomes corresponding to all the spinal nerve roots are shown in Fig. 6.2. With spinal cord disease, a cardinal physical sign is the presence of a **sensory level**. Thus, for example, a patient may have impaired cutaneous sensation in all dermatomes below T10 (Fig. 6.1d). As discussed in Chapter 15, this does not necessarily mean that the level of the lesion in the spinal cord is at T10, but rather that it is anywhere at *or above* that level. Hence, sensory levels generally have less localizing value than reflex or motor levels (Chapter 5).

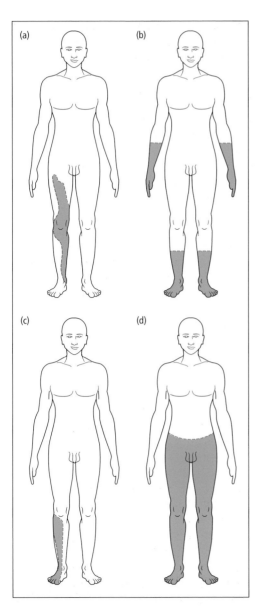

Figure 6.1 Patterns of sensory loss. (a) Mononeuropathy – isolated damage to an individual peripheral nerve, in this example a complete lesion of the right femoral nerve; (b) polyneuropathy – 'glove-and-stocking' distribution of impairment; (c) dermatomal – sensory loss corresponding to the cutaneous distribution of a spinal nerve root, in this case right L5; (d) sensory level – characteristic of spinal cord lesions.

Higher sensory function

Patients with disease of the parietal cortex may have relatively subtle sensory deficits, not necessarily detected by testing the crude modalities of sensation. For such patients, other sensory tests are available, as follows.

Two-point discrimination

Using a pair of dividers, a patient's ability to discriminate between the application of one point or both points simultaneously can be determined. The minimum distance at which the simultaneous application of both points is detectable can then be ascertained with the patient's eyes shut. This distance varies according to the site on the body where it is being tested, but is normally 2–3 mm on the finger pulps. Although the distance of two-point discrimination may increase with disease of lower sensory pathways, the test is particularly valuable in patients with higher sensory deficits.

Sensory inattention

When a sensory stimulus is simultaneously applied to both sides of the body, patients with parietal cortical disease, particularly of the non-dominant lobe, may fail to report the stimulus on the side contralateral to the site of damage. This phenomenon is allied to visual inattention (Chapter 4) and to the **neglect** of the left side of the body, indeed the left side of the world, sometimes seen in patients with non-dominant, i.e. usually right-sided, parietal lobe damage (Chapter 3).

Agraphaesthesia

Inability to identify numbers drawn by the examiner on the patient's palm, with the patient's eyes shut.

Astereognosis

Inability to identify objects in three dimensions, e.g. distinguishing by touch alone between coins placed by the examiner in the patient's hand.

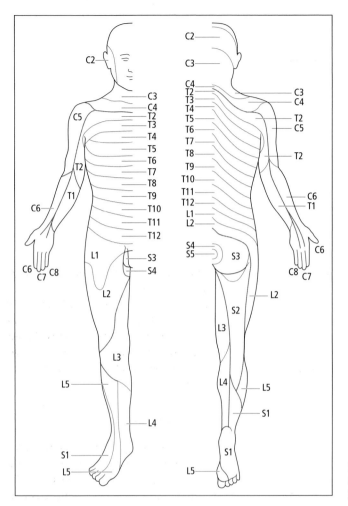

Figure 6.2 Approximate distribution of the dermatomes on the anterior and posterior aspects of the body.

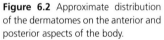

Key points

- The modalities of sensation amenable to routine clinical testing are joint position, vibration, touch and pressure, and pain and temperature
- Sensory signs elicited in the absence of symptoms are of dubious significance
- The sensory examination is always subjective
- Patterns of sensory loss may point to particular disorders, e.g. 'glove-and-stocking' loss in peripheral neuropathy, sensory level in spinal cord disease

Chapter 7

Autonomic function

The autonomic nervous system is concerned with the involuntary control of visceral and glandular function. Disturbances of its parasympathetic and/or sympathetic components may affect several clinically important sites:

- pupils (Chapter 4),
- control of blood pressure and heart rate,
- bladder, bowel and sexual function,
- sweating, lacrimation, salivation.

Clinical features

Blood pressure

Failure to maintain blood pressure on assuming an upright posture may present with lightheadedness, dizziness, or even syncope (Chapter 2), and other non-specific symptoms (e.g., blurred vision, fatigue, nausea, head and neck pain). It may also be asymptomatic. In all symptomatic cases, there is a relationship to the assumption of an erect posture or following head-up tilt.

Orthostatic hypotension is defined as a fall of systolic blood pressure of at least 20 mm Hg or diastolic blood pressure of at least 10 mm Hg within 3 minutes of standing. Typically, the

Lecture Notes: Neurology, 9th edition. By Lionel Ginsberg.
Published 2010 by Blackwell Publishing.

normal compensatory increase in pulse rate on standing is also absent.

Although postural hypotension of this degree may signify underlying disease of the autonomic nervous system (**autonomic failure**), confounding factors may produce a similar picture, particularly the overzealous use of antihypertensive drugs in the elderly.

Sphincter dysfunction

Broadly speaking, neurogenic bladder dysfunction falls into two main categories, analogous to upper and lower motor neurone (UMN and LMN) lesions affecting striated muscle. Thus, damage to the equivalent of the LMN for the bladder (S2, 3 and 4 parasympathetic fibres), either at their origin in the lower spinal cord ('conus') or in the cauda equina or pelvis, interrupts the normal reflex arc and the bladder fills but is unable to empty properly (urinary retention ultimately with **overflow** incontinence). The bladder becomes palpable and may be tender, depending on whether the afferent fibres are also affected. Infection is common.

Damage to the equivalent of the UMN for the bladder, as a result of incomplete lesions higher in the spinal cord, with loss of supraspinal inhibition, renders the muscle wall of the bladder increasingly irritable (**detrusor instability**). Patients develop urgency and frequency of micturition, ultimately with **urge** incontinence of urine. Although this broad subdivision is conceptually useful, the clinical picture is often mixed and also complicated by the voluntary control mechanisms of the bladder.

Bowel dysfunction apart from constipation is a late feature of spinal cord disease, but may occur at presentation with lesions of the cauda equina, with absolute constipation, faecal impaction and ultimately overflow incontinence of faeces.

More widespread damage to the innervation of the gastrointestinal tract, as may occur in diabetes mellitus, produces a mixture of abnormalities of gut function, including:
- failure of gastric emptying (**gastroparesis**) with distension, pain, nausea and vomiting;
- abnormal intestinal motility, either reduced (again with abdominal pain and vomiting – **pseudo-obstruction**) or increased (with diarrhoea, including nocturnally, and faecal incontinence).

Sexual dysfunction in men, particularly erectile impotence, is a common accompaniment of autonomic failure.

Other symptoms and signs

Patients may be aware of reduced or absent sweating (**anhidrosis**). Dry eyes and a dry mouth are more often due to disease of the effector organs themselves (lacrimal and salivary glands), as in Sjögren's syndrome, or due to use of anticholinergic drugs, than impaired autonomic innervation. However, some patients with **paraneoplastic** disorders, e.g. Lambert–Eaton myasthenic syndrome (Chapters 17 and 19), experience a dry mouth as a result of involvement of the autonomic nervous system.

Investigations

In addition to bedside tests, e.g. lying and standing blood pressure, more sophisticated **autonomic function tests** are available:
- Cardiovascular
  - blood pressure response to tilt,
  - loss of normal beat-to-beat variation in heart rate (sinus arrhythmia) detected by measuring R–R interval on ECG,

- loss of reflex bradycardia to Valsalva manoeuvre (straining by forced expiration against closed glottis);
- Bladder
- **urodynamic** studies (monitoring intravesical pressure as a function of filling) often in combination with dynamic imaging (**video-cystometrogram**) and **electromyography** (Chapter 8) of the bladder sphincter.

Specific conditions

Autonomic failure may rarely be inherited (familial dysautonomia: Riley–Day syndrome) or may arise as a result of disease at several sites in the nervous system, as follows.

Central nervous system

Pure autonomic failure, manifesting predominantly with orthostatic hypotension, may occur without other neurological features. But autonomic failure may also develop in a minority of patients with Parkinson's disease (Chapter 12) and also in **multiple system atrophy**. The latter is a progressive disorder characterized by:
- Parkinsonian features,
- cerebellar and/or UMN signs,
- autonomic dysfunction, particularly orthostatic hypotension, impotence and urinary retention or incontinence.

These and other features may occur in various combinations (Chapter 12). When autonomic failure predominates, the condition is often termed **Shy–Drager syndrome**.

Hypothalamus

Within the central nervous system (CNS), the hypothalamus acts as a higher integrating centre of sympathetic and parasympathetic activity. Patients with rare structural lesions, e.g. tumours, in this region may develop disorders of appetite, thirst, sleep and temperature control, along with disturbances of pituitary regulation.

Peripheral nerves

Inflammatory or metabolic damage to the peripheral nerves, resulting in a **polyneuropathy**, may affect autonomic as well as sensory and motor fibres. In the Guillain–Barré syndrome (Chapter 20), patients may have labile blood pressure and cardiac dysrhythmias in addition to the other potentially life-threatening aspects of this condition. Other causes of a polyneuropathy where autonomic failure may be a dominant feature include (commonly) diabetes mellitus and (rarely) amyloidosis.

Sympathetic dysfunction and pain

There is an incompletely understood relationship between sympathetic nerve fibres and pain afferents, which are similarly small in diameter and unmyelinated. Thus, partial peripheral nerve trauma may lead to a chronic neurogenic pain syndrome with sympathetic accompaniments, including shiny, red, dry skin with hair loss, some swelling and poor wound healing in the affected limb. When this combination affects the distribution of a particular nerve or root, it is termed **causalgia**. When the anatomical basis is less clear-cut, the term **reflex sympathetic dystrophy** or complex regional pain syndrome is used.

Treatment

• **Symptomatic postural hypotension** may be managed by the patient sleeping in a bed with a head-up tilt. Fludrocortisone, a mineralocorticoid, may also be beneficial, but many patients respond poorly to this and other drugs that have been tried, such as indomethacin.

• **Bladder hyperreflexia** with detrusor instability may respond to anticholinergic drugs, e.g. oxybutynin or tolterodine.

• **Chronic retention of urine** may require intermittent self-catheterization. Patients with mixed bladder disturbances may need both intermittent self-catheterization and anticholinergics. Infection must be treated early.

• **Erectile impotence** may respond to intracorporeal injection of papaverine or prostaglandins, or to use of a vacuum device. Oral medication is also now available (sildenafil and related drugs).

• **Causalgia** and related chronic regional pain syndromes may respond to sympathectomy to the affected limb.

Key points

• Postural hypotension is an important manifestation of autonomic failure, readily assessed at the bedside
• Neurogenic bladder dysfunction may be subdivided into the equivalent of upper and lower motor neurone patterns, though this is a simplification
• Autonomic failure may complicate peripheral neuropathy (as commonly seen in diabetes mellitus) or may arise centrally (as in multiple system atrophy)

Chapter 8

Investigating the patient

The importance of accurate history-taking and physical examination in reaching a neurological diagnosis cannot be overstated. However, many patients require specialist investigation for a definitive diagnosis, or at least to provide laboratory support for clinical suspicions.

Neuroimaging

Some of the greatest advances in neurological investigation in the last 35 years have involved brain and spinal imaging, to the extent that some time-honoured radiological techniques have been virtually abandoned in favour of newer non-invasive high-resolution technology.

Plain X-rays

Plain radiographs of skull and spine (Fig. 8.1) now have limited usefulness beyond the investigation of acute trauma, i.e. to detect a fracture.

Computed tomographic (CT) scanning

CT scanning remains the primary investigation of choice for many intracranial lesions and has a role in spinal imaging. The technique relies on the reconstruction of tomographic images (a se-

ries of horizontal slices) resulting from the passage of X-rays through the body in multiple directions. Examples of normal CT scans of the head are shown in Fig. 8.2. Further refinement of the images is provided by administration of an intravenous iodine-containing contrast medium, which highlights ('**enhances**') areas of increased vascularity or regions where there is breakdown of the blood–brain barrier.

Abnormalities detectable on CT scans include high-density areas, indicating blood or calcium, and low or mixed density seen in many other pathological processes – examples of abnormal scans are given in the second part of this book in the context of the relevant clinical condition. One important property of any lesion seen on CT cranial scan is whether it exerts **mass effect**, as evidenced by compression of the ventricles or shift of midline structures.

Magnetic resonance imaging (MRI)

MRI has several advantages over CT scanning. Unlike the latter, it does not depend on X-rays, but rather on the response of a tissue's protons in a strong magnetic field to the effects of a brief radiofrequency pulse. After the pulse, displaced protons realign with the magnetic field, and the rate of realignment, along with other features including the proton density, gives information about physical properties of the tissue, notably its water

Lecture Notes: Neurology, 9th edition. By Lionel Ginsberg. Published 2010 by Blackwell Publishing.

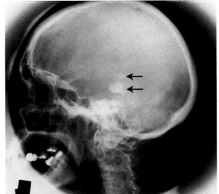

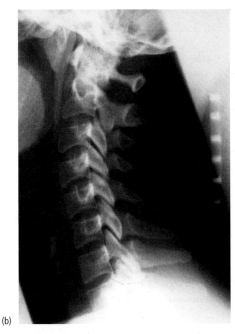

Figure 8.1 Plain radiographs of skull and spine. (a) Normal lateral skull radiograph – note prominent calcification of pineal gland and choroid plexus in this example (upper and lower arrows, respectively); (b) normal lateral radiograph of the cervical spine.

content. This information may be reconstructed by a computer to give images in any plane, i.e. sagittal and coronal images as well as axial scans are obtained with greater ease and resolution than is possible with CT scanning. Examples of normal MR scans are shown in Fig. 8.3. The technique provides information on regions less well seen with CT scanning, e.g. the posterior cranial fossa and

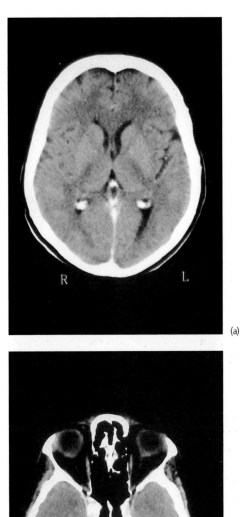

Figure 8.2 Normal CT cranial scans showing (a) the cerebral hemispheres and (b) the temporal lobes and posterior fossa.

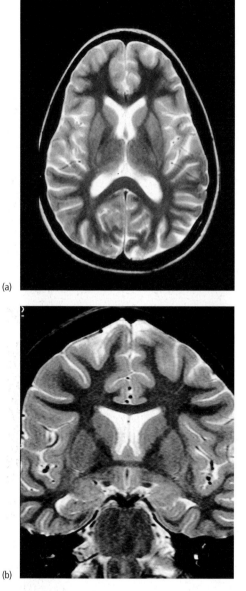

(a)

(b)

Figure 8.3 Normal MR scans of the brain. (a) Axial and (b) coronal sections.

Invasive studies

Myelography

Before the advent of spinal MRI, imaging of the spinal cord and nerve roots was achieved using a water-soluble contrast medium injected into the subarachnoid space by lumbar puncture (see below). Flow of contrast up the spinal canal is regulated on a tilting table, the patient being directly screened using an image intensifier throughout the procedure. Radiographs are taken of relevant segments of the spine (Fig. 8.4). Myelography is now used only rarely, for example in patients where MRI is contraindicated, such as individuals with cardiac pacemakers.

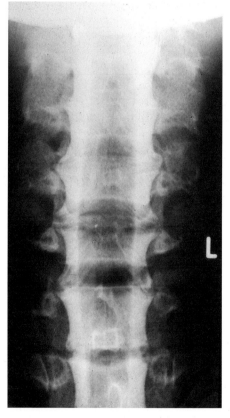

Figure 8.4 Normal cervical myelogram (anteroposterior view). The intrathecal contrast medium outlines the normal expansion of the cervical spinal cord.

the spine, and has been especially helpful in the investigation of diseases of white matter (Chapter 16). Again, additional refinement is provided by the use of an intravenous contrast medium, this time based on the rare earth **gadolinium**.

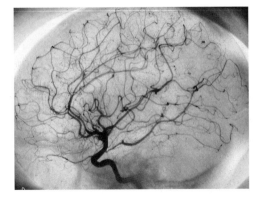

Figure 8.5 Normal internal carotid arteriogram.

Angiography

Formal imaging of the carotid and vertebral circulations is achieved using contrast medium injected into the relevant artery via a catheter introduced into the body usually through the femoral artery and threaded up the vascular tree to the neck vessels with the aid of an image intensifier. A series of radiographs is taken, showing contrast first outlining the branches of the carotid or vertebral arteries (clinically the most important phase, Fig. 8.5) and then the capillary and venous circulations. Similar techniques may be used to study the spinal circulation, though the latter procedure is particularly laborious and technically demanding, as so many supplying vessels have to be catheterized. Spinal angiography is generally conducted under general anaesthesia, but this is not usually necessary for the cranial circulation.

Numerous approaches have been developed to avoid the risks, albeit small, of formal angiography (i.e., cerebral or spinal ischaemia as a result of embolism, hypotension or vasospasm):

• **Digital subtraction angiography** (DSA) – contrast medium may be injected intravenously with this technique. Computerized **subtraction** of the pre-contrast from the post-contrast image allows display of the vessels in virtual isolation (Fig. 8.6a). This technique has now been largely superseded by MR and CT angiography.

• **MR angiography** – blood vessels may be delineated using MR techniques (Fig. 8.6b), as they

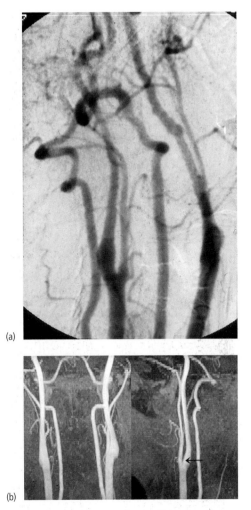

(a)

(b)

Figure 8.6 (a) Intravenous DSA and (b) MR angiography – both of the neck vessels. The MR angiogram shows the vessels in an anteroposterior (left) and lateral (right) view. The internal carotid artery is arrowed in the lateral view.

typically produce a low signal because of intraluminal blood flow ('flow void').

• **CT angiography** – high-resolution CT scanning with intravenous contrast and subtraction techniques now also permits study of vascular anatomy.

Interventional neuroradiology

Needle aspiration and biopsy of lesions, particularly in the spinal region, may be aided by CT or MR guidance.

Interventional methods also have a therapeutic role in the context of intracranial aneurysms and vascular malformations (Chapter 11).

Functional imaging

Most of the techniques described in this chapter have been concerned with the structure of the CNS. More recently, however, methods for imaging brain function have been developed, albeit largely in a research setting. In particular, **positron emission tomography** (PET) has yielded information on cerebral blood flow and volume, oxygen and glucose metabolic rates, and even on neurotransmitter function, particularly in dopaminergic pathways. The technique relies on the detection of photons released by collisions between positrons emitted by administered radionuclides (bound to molecules of biological interest) and electrons in the brain tissue. Computerized reconstruction of these events detected by a specialized camera yields brain images, with spatial resolution of the particular function being studied. Measurements may be made at rest or with activation, e.g. sensory stimulation or motor action.

Various factors have limited the application of PET as a diagnostic tool beyond specialist centres. In particular, the short half-life of most positron-emitting radionuclides means there must be a cyclotron near the site of scanning. This problem has been avoided with **single-photon-emission computed tomography** (SPECT), which utilizes gamma-emitting radionuclides. However, the spatial resolution of SPECT is inferior to that of PET. More recently, brain function has been investigated with functional MRI and **in vivo MR spectroscopy**.

Clinical neurophysiology

Electroencephalography (EEG)

The spontaneous electrical activity of the brain is recorded via scalp electrodes in a routine EEG (see Fig. 10.1, p. 75). An 8- or 16-channel tracing

Table 8.1 Normal EEG rhythms.

Rhythm	Frequency (Hz)	Characteristics
Alpha	8–13	Symmetrical, present posteriorly with eyes closed, disappears with eye-opening
Beta	> 13	Symmetrical, frontal, unaffected by eye-opening
Theta	4–8	Seen in children and adolescents, frontal and temporal predominance
Delta	< 4	

shows changes in electrical potential with time, usually between pairs of adjacent electrodes. The arrangement of electrodes on the scalp ('montage') permits all major areas of cerebral cortex to be electrically sampled.

Normal EEG rhythms are summarized in Table 8.1. In disease, abnormalities include:
- generalized slowing – as seen in a metabolic encephalopathy (Chapter 19) or encephalitis (Chapter 14),
- focal excess slow activity – indicating a unilateral structural lesion,
- paroxysmal high-voltage discharges ('spikes' and sharp waves) (focal or generalized), supporting a diagnosis of epilepsy (Chapter 10).

Many patients with epilepsy have a normal resting EEG between attacks. The diagnostic yield of this investigation can be increased by stressing the patient during the recording, e.g. by asking them to hyperventilate or by photic stimulation with a flashing light. In addition, prolonged recordings may be helpful, particularly after overnight **sleep deprivation** or induction of sleep with a barbiturate. In specialist centres, EEG recording is possible in ambulant patients with simultaneous video recording to correlate clinical events with electrical changes (**videotelemetry**).

Evoked potentials

Sensory stimulation will produce an electrical signal in the relevant area of the cerebral cortex. This minute response is normally lost in the background electrical activity, but it can be revealed by averaging techniques which remove 'noise', the evoked potential being 'time-locked' to the stimulus.

Visual evoked potentials are recorded after retinal stimulation with stroboscopic flashes, or an alternating chequerboard pattern. A signal is obtained using EEG electrodes over the occipital region. This potential is reduced in many ocular conditions, and may be delayed by optic nerve disease (Chapter 16).

Brainstem auditory evoked potentials and **somatosensory evoked potentials** are elicited by audible 'clicks' and electrical stimulation of a peripheral nerve (e.g., the median), respectively. Recordings are made with surface electrodes over the mastoid and vertex for the former, and neck and parietal region for the latter. Somatosensory evoked potentials provide an estimate of **central conduction time** by comparing the latency of the response recorded at the neck (spinal cord) with that over the parietal cortex. Similarly, **central motor conduction time** may be obtained by comparing the latency to a muscle response following stimulation of the motor cortex (usually with an external magnet) with that following an external electrical stimulus to the spinal cord, applied to the neck. The clinical usefulness of these techniques has declined in recent years with advances in neuroimaging.

Electromyography (EMG) and nerve conduction studies

Diseases of the peripheral nervous system, neuromuscular junction and muscle are all amenable to electrodiagnostic investigation.

EMG involves insertion of a **concentric needle electrode** into a muscle to record its electrical activity directly, both at rest and on contraction. The principal aim of such studies is to distinguish between primary muscle disease (**myopathy**) and EMG abnormalities that are secondary to denervation, i.e. indicative of a **neurogenic** disorder.

Nerve conduction studies involve electrical stimulation of a nerve and measurement of several variables, including the **conduction velocity** (both motor and sensory) and **amplitude** of the action potential (Fig. 8.7). Damage to the peripheral nerves (**neuropathy** – Chapter 17) may primarily involve the axons themselves, in which case the electrodiagnostic hallmark is a reduction in the amplitude of the action potential. Alternatively, if the primary site of damage is the myelin sheath (**demyelinating** vs. **axonal** neuropathy), the dominant feature in nerve conduction studies is a reduction in conduction velocity. Sometimes, a mixed picture is seen.

Other techniques aid diagnosis of neuromuscular junction disorders. Thus, when a motor nerve is subjected to **repetitive stimulation**, the resulting muscle action potential normally has a constant amplitude (unless the stimulus frequency is very high). In myasthenia gravis (Chapter 17) the response rapidly fatigues, as evidenced by a **decrement** in amplitude. Interestingly, other disorders of neuromuscular transmission (specifically the Lambert–Eaton myasthenic syndrome – Chapters 17 and 19) may be associated with an **incremental** response to repetitive stimulation. Neuromuscular junction defects may also be analysed by sophisticated EMG methods, using finer needle electrodes with a smaller recording surface than usual (**single-fibre EMG**).

Fluids and tissues

Cerebrospinal fluid (CSF)

The normal pressure and constituents of CSF are summarized in Table 8.2. In addition to these basic characteristics, a sample of CSF obtained at **lumbar puncture** (Fig. 8.8) may be analysed as follows:

- Bacteriology
  - Gram stain and culture,
  - Ziehl–Neelsen stain and culture for tubercle bacillus,
  - serological tests for syphilis;

Chapter 9

Headache and facial pain

Headaches may be subdivided into:
- those with a defined pathophysiological basis ('secondary' headaches),
- those of uncertain pathogenesis ('primary' headache syndromes).

Headaches with a defined pathophysiological basis may represent a threat to the patient's life, vision or other neurological function. Primary headache syndromes are generally more benign (and, in the case of migraine and tension-type headache, much more common) but are still a significant source of morbidity.

Headaches with a defined pathophysiological basis

Disorders of intracranial pressure

The headache of raised intracranial pressure, e.g. caused by cerebral tumour, is characteristically present on waking or indeed may wake the patient at night. It may improve later in the day. Occipital 'bursting' pain is of particular significance. The headache may be exacerbated by sneezing, straining, bending, lifting or lying down, all of which may raise intracranial pressure further. Patients with headache caused by an intracranial tu-

mour generally have a short history – days, weeks or at most months. There is usually a crescendo quality to the symptom, the pain becoming increasingly severe and persistent, and ultimately occurring daily, without fail (Fig. 1.1). There may be associated nausea and vomiting. **Effortless vomiting,** with or without associated nausea, is a symptom of a mass in the posterior fossa, close to the fourth ventricle, irritating the vomiting centre.

Although patients with occipital morning pain but no neurological signs generally warrant a CT scan to exclude an intracranial mass, only a small minority will prove to have a brain tumour. Conversely, patients with brain tumours only rarely present with headache alone. The headache may be a relatively mild symptom, other neurological features predominating. More definitive symptoms and signs of raised intracranial pressure as a result of mass lesions and other causes are described in Chapter 13.

Headaches may also signify low intracranial pressure. The hallmark of such headaches is their relation to posture, pain being rapidly relieved by lying down. Although such headaches have long been an acknowledged consequence of lumbar puncture (Chapter 8), **spontaneous low-pressure headache** is an increasingly recognized phenomenon.

Lecture Notes: Neurology, 9th edition. By Lionel Ginsberg. Published 2010 by Blackwell Publishing.

Idiopathic ('benign') intracranial hypertension

This condition typically occurs in young, obese women. There are symptoms and signs of raised intracranial pressure but no mass lesion is identified on cranial imaging with CT or MR. The pathophysiology is incompletely understood but may involve impaired CSF absorption.

Patients present with morning headache, vomiting and sometimes visual disturbance – typically diplopia and **visual obscurations** (sudden, transient bilateral visual loss with changes in posture). Tinnitus is also a common symptom. Examination reveals bilateral papilloedema. Unilateral or bilateral sixth nerve palsies may also be present as a 'false localizing sign' of raised intracranial pressure (Chapter 4), but no other focal neurological signs are found. CT scanning of the brain excludes a mass lesion and reveals ventricles of normal or small size (as opposed to hydrocephalus – Chapter 13). CSF examination by lumbar puncture (safe after an intracranial mass has been excluded on imaging) confirms raised pressure (often very high, greater than 40 cm of CSF) with normal CSF contents.

The condition may be self-limiting, resolving completely with weight loss and after one or a few lumbar punctures. In some patients, however, it is more chronic and there is a threat to vision from secondary optic atrophy. In these instances, medical treatment with the carbonic anhydrase inhibitor acetazolamide, other diuretics, e.g. chlortalidone, or corticosteroids may be successful. But surgical intervention may be required either to drain CSF via a lumboperitoneal shunt or to protect the optic nerve via fenestration procedures (optic nerve sheath incision).

The threat to vision renders the term *benign* intracranial hypertension somewhat inappropriate, but other attempts to name the condition, e.g. **pseudotumour cerebri**, have proved equally awkward. By definition, benign intracranial hypertension is idiopathic, but a similar syndrome may be symptomatic of:

- intracranial venous sinus thrombosis (Chapter 11),
- hypervitaminosis A,
- disturbances of calcium metabolism,
- systemic lupus erythematosus,
- drugs, including tetracyclines and corticosteroids (paradoxically, as the latter are also used to treat the condition).

Meningeal irritation

Meningism or irritation of the meninges, e.g. by inflammatory processes (as in acute meningitis, Chapter 14) or blood (subarachnoid haemorrhage, Chapter 11), characteristically produces severe global or occipital headache with vomiting, exacerbation of symptoms by bright lights (photophobia) and neck stiffness (**nuchal rigidity**).

In subarachnoid haemorrhage, the pain is usually very sudden in onset (within seconds) and severe, and the patient may lose consciousness. In bacterial meningitis, the headache is also acute in onset, but usually worsening over minutes or hours.

Nuchal rigidity is assessed by determining the patient's resistance to passive neck flexion. Meningism may also be demonstrated by **Kernig's sign** (pain and resistance to passive knee extension with the hip flexed). In some patients, particularly children, nuchal rigidity may be due to a posterior fossa mass rather than a diffuse meningeal process, but in such individuals Kernig's sign is usually negative.

Giant cell arteritis (cranial arteritis, temporal arteritis)

This is an important condition in patients older than 50 years. Granulomatous inflammatory changes (with giant cells) are present in branches of the external carotid artery, particularly the superficial temporal vessels, but also elsewhere, including intracranial vessels and the blood supply to the optic nerve head. The blood vessels show narrowing of the lumen, which may become occluded with thrombus. The aetiology is uncertain, but viral infection and autoimmunity have been implicated.

Patients usually present with headache which may be non-specific but may localize to the temples, where there may also be tenderness. Scalp tenderness may become apparent when patients attempt to comb their hair. Pain on chewing is attributed to impairment of blood supply to the muscles of mastication (**intermittent claudication of the jaw**). The temporal arteries may become swollen and non-pulsatile; rarely skin ulceration occurs.

Transient loss of vision in one eye (**amaurosis fugax**) is an ominous symptom, the patient being at risk of permanent monocular or indeed complete blindness. Diplopia may result from third or sixth nerve involvement.

Constitutional symptoms include low-grade fever, night sweats, shoulder and/or pelvic girdle pains, malaise, anorexia and weight loss. Evidence of more generalized arteritis includes disturbance of liver function, rarely a peripheral neuropathy, and involvement of intracranial vessels, i.e. stroke, particularly in vertebrobasilar territory.

Because of the threat to vision and other neurological consequences, early diagnosis and treatment are essential. Salient investigations are:
- ESR often grossly elevated (greater than 100 mm/h), the C-reactive protein level will also be high;
- other blood tests which may reveal a normochromic, normocytic anaemia and abnormal liver function tests, particularly raised alkaline phosphatase;
- temporal artery biopsy.

Though the last investigation is important if positive, a negative biopsy does not exclude giant cell arteritis (because the artery may not be uniformly involved histologically along its length, i.e. there may be '**skip lesions**') and patients may need to be treated on clinical grounds alone.

If giant cell arteritis is suspected, patients should be treated urgently with intravenous hydrocortisone once blood has been taken for ESR, i.e. before the biopsy (diagnostic histological changes may still be seen on biopsy a week or more after commencing steroids). Fortunately, the condition is highly sensitive to corticosteroids, though high doses (40–60 mg daily of prednisolone) are ini-

tially required. A rapid response to steroids is helpful diagnostically, patients often feeling dramatically better within 24–48 hours. The dose is then gradually tapered down, according to the patient's symptoms and ESR, but treatment for 18 months to 2 years is usually required. The allied condition of **polymyalgia rheumatica,** characterized by girdle pains and morning stiffness with some constitutional upset but without the cranial manifestations of giant cell arteritis, is also dramatically responsive to corticosteroids, often in lower dosage (7.5–15 mg daily of prednisolone).

Other causes

Headache often accompanies stroke, especially when caused by haemorrhage, intracranial venous sinus thrombosis or arterial dissection (Chapter 11). Metabolic disturbances, e.g. hypoxia, hypercapnia and hypoglycaemia, can trigger headache, as can vasoactive drugs and other substances (such as alcohol, monosodium glutamate, nitrites and nitrates). Local extracranial causes of headache and facial pain are listed at the end of this chapter.

Primary headache syndromes

Migraine

Definition, epidemiology and causation

Migraine is a periodic disorder characterized by unilateral (or sometimes bilateral) headache, which may be associated with vomiting and visual disturbance.

It is a common condition, more than 10% of the general population experiencing at least one migraine attack in their lifetime. Migraine may develop at any age, but onset typically is in the teens or twenties, and women are more often affected. A family history of migraine is present in the majority of patients. Many individuals with travel sickness and cyclical vomiting in childhood subsequently develop migraine. There is also a relationship to hypertension and head injury.

The underlying pathophysiology is obscure, but initial neurological symptoms – the **aura** (visual, sensory and other phenomena) – have traditionally been attributed to a phase of intracerebral vasoconstriction (this is almost certainly a simplification; the aura more probably corresponds to a spreading wave of depolarization across the cerebral cortex). Subsequent vasodilatation, particularly of extracerebral vessels in the scalp and dura, may be responsible for the headache. There is pharmacological evidence for involvement of serotoninergic (5-HT) pathways along with vasoactive neuropeptides. Genetic studies of families with hemiplegic migraine (see below) have recently indicated a role for calcium channels in the pathogenesis. Various factors may trigger migraine attacks, including:

- stress, particularly after the stress is over, e.g. at weekends and holidays;
- physical exercise;
- diet – alcohol; occasionally specific dietary triggers can be identified, e.g. cheese, chocolate, red wine;
- hormones – the onset of migraine may follow the menarche, and symptoms may also increase in severity around the menopause. Attacks may be related to menstruation.

Clinical features

Several syndromes are recognized, as described below.

Migraine with aura (classical migraine)

The patient may experience vague prodromal symptoms for hours preceding an attack, including drowsiness, mood changes, hunger or anorexia. The classical attack begins with the aura. Visual symptoms include expanding scotomata, which may scintillate (**teichopsia**). Crenated or castellated patterns may appear (**fortification spectra**). A homonymous hemianopia or complete blindness may result. Sensory symptoms are less common, but unilateral numbness and paraesthesiae may affect the face, arm and/or leg. Dysphasia and limb weakness are rare.

The aura generally resolves after 15–20 minutes (it may last as long as an hour), at which stage headache supervenes, though in some patients,

headache and focal neurological symptoms coexist. The headache of migraine is typically unilateral and periorbital, often contralateral to the side of the hemianopia. Pain is throbbing in quality and may be exacerbated by coughing, straining or bending (**jolt phenomenon**). It lasts several hours (generally between 4 and 72 hours). Patients prefer to lie in a darkened room and may gain relief from sleep. Associated symptoms include photophobia, nausea, vomiting, pallor and diuresis.

Migraine without aura (common migraine)

In this case, the aura is absent but patients may experience vague prodromal symptoms. Headache may be present on waking but is otherwise similar to that of classical migraine.

Basilar migraine (Bickerstaff variant)

This syndrome, which particularly affects teenage female patients, is characterized by prominent features suggestive of vertebrobasilar ischaemia during the aura, including vertigo, diplopia, dysarthria, ataxia and syncope.

Hemiplegic and ophthalmoplegic migraine

These rare syndromes, in which migrainous headaches are accompanied by hemiplegia or ophthalmoplegia, with focal neurological signs persisting for days or weeks, should be diagnosed only after structural causes, e.g. aneurysm, have been excluded.

Diagnosis

Migraine is diagnosed almost exclusively on the history, the periodicity of attacks being particularly important. Patients have episodes of headache usually lasting less than 3 days and then pain-free periods varying from days to months. Continuous headache week after week is unlikely to be due to straightforward migraine, though rarely a **status migrainosus** may develop. Neurological examination is normal (except during an attack of hemiplegic or ophthalmoplegic migraine, or unless migrainous cerebral infarction has occurred), thereby helping to differentiate migraine from more sinister underlying causes of headache, e.g. raised intracranial pressure. The rare finding of a **cranial bruit** should alert the physician to the remote possibility of migraine being associated with a vascular malformation of the brain.

In general, the differential diagnosis of transient focal neurological symptoms is:

- migraine,
- transient cerebral ischaemia,
- epilepsy.

Migraine can usually be distinguished from the other two possibilities by the rate of spread of symptoms, which is much slower than in an epileptic or transient ischaemic attack (minutes rather than seconds or less), and by the presence of associated symptoms.

Focal neurological features always recurring on the same side may prompt brain imaging to exclude an underlying lesion, but strict unilaterality is much more likely to be due to migraine in the context of an otherwise appropriate history than any other cause.

Management

Acute attack

Patients benefit from lying in a darkened room and from sleep. Simple soluble analgesics, e.g. paracetamol or aspirin, should be taken in combination with an antiemetic. Episodes unresponsive to such measures may be treated with **ergotamine**, a potent vasoconstrictor (used rarely nowadays), or one of the **triptans**, such as **sumatriptan**, a selective 5-HT$_1$ receptor agonist, which may be given subcutaneously, intranasally or orally. Both drugs have disadvantages. Ergot alkaloids may cause acute poisoning (**ergotism**), with vomiting, muscle pain and weakness, paraesthesiae in the extremities, chest pain, pruritus and cardiac dysrhythmias. Chronic excessive use may lead to gangrene, hence ergotamine is contraindicated in peripheral vascular disease. Sumatriptan interacts with ergotamine, monoamine oxidase inhibitors, selective 5-HT reuptake inhibitors and lithium. Combined use of these drugs is contraindicated, as is the use of sumatriptan or ergotamine in patients with ischaemic heart disease.

Prophylaxis

Clear-cut dietary triggers should be avoided. Oestrogen-containing preparations, e.g. oral contraceptives and hormone replacement therapy, should be used with caution in migraine sufferers, as they may exacerbate migrainous tendencies. Patients with frequent attacks, i.e. more than one per month, may warrant treatment with prophylactic drugs. The first-line agents are **propranolol** and other **beta-blockers,** and **pizotifen**, a 5-HT$_2$ receptor antagonist. Treatment with either a beta-blocker or pizotifen for 3–6 months may be sufficient to reduce the frequency of attacks, without recurrence on drug withdrawal. Beta-blockers are contraindicated in uncontrolled heart failure, obstructive airways disease, severe peripheral vascular disease and cardiac bradyarrhythmias. The main side effects of pizotifen are drowsiness and weight gain; anticholinergic effects also limit its use in patients with glaucoma and urinary retention.

Other prophylactic drugs include **sodium valproate, verapamil, topiramate** and **methysergide**. Use of the last (another 5-HT receptor antagonist) should be restricted to patients with severe and frequent migraines, unresponsive to other agents, and is best used under hospital supervision in view of the risk of severe side effects, particularly the development of **retroperitoneal fibrosis**. Tricyclic antidepressants, e.g. amitriptyline, and related drugs, e.g. dosulepin, are beneficial in migraine prophylaxis, particularly in patients who have coexistent tension-type headache (see below).

Cluster headache

Despite also being characterized by unilateral headache, this syndrome is distinct from migraine, though the two conditions may coexist. Histaminergic and other humoral mechanisms are thought to underlie the autonomic accompaniments of the headache.

Patients are usually male, and the age of onset is 20–60 years. Severe attacks of pain around one eye (always the same side) characteristically last 20–120 minutes and may recur several times a day, often waking the patient more than once at night. Alcohol may precipitate an attack. This pattern continues for days, weeks or months, and the patient may then be symptom-free for many weeks, months or even years, hence the disorder's name. Unlike migraine, patients with cluster headache are often restless during an attack and may appear red rather than pale. More pronounced autonomic accompaniments of the pain include conjunctival injection, lacrimation and nasal discharge or congestion. A full-blown **Horner's syndrome** may develop and persist after the attack. These phenomena are all unilateral, occurring on the side of the pain.

Treatment to abolish a cluster includes the use of high-flow 100% oxygen, ergotamine (best in suppository form at bedtime in combination with caffeine), sumatriptan or corticosteroids (e.g., a 2-week reducing course of prednisolone or dexamethasone). Longer-term treatment to prevent recurrence of a cluster may involve use of methysergide, verapamil or pizotifen. Lithium is particularly helpful if the clusters become more chronic but blood levels must be monitored, as with its use in affective disorders.

Several other conditions have been described in which unilateral headache and/or facial pain are associated with autonomic features. Some of these rare 'trigeminal–autonomic' syndromes are strikingly responsive to indometacin.

Tension-type headache

This very common condition remains of unknown cause though abnormal contraction of muscles of the head and neck has been invoked as one putative mechanism. Muscle contraction may be triggered by psychogenic factors, i.e. anxiety or depression, or by local disease of the head and neck, e.g. cervical spondylosis or dental malocclusion. Descriptions of the headache vary from dull pain at various sites, to a global pressure sensation, to the feeling of a tight band around the head. More exotic and bizarre descriptions may point to a psychogenic basis in some patients. There are no associated symptoms, and neurological

examination is normal. Migraine and tension-type headache frequently coexist.

Treatment includes reassurance that there is no sinister underlying cause. A 3–6-month course of a tricyclic or related compound, e.g. amitriptyline or dosulepin, may be helpful if tension-type headache is frequent or persistent. This may also aid analgesic withdrawal (see below). Other patients may benefit from advice from a physiotherapist, including relaxation exercises, or psychotherapy (stress management).

Chronic daily headache

Headache occurring on 15 or more days per month is termed chronic daily headache. Causes include secondary headache syndromes (see above), chronic tension-type headache and 'transformed' migraine. In the last condition, the normal periodicity of migraine is lost, but other migrainous features may persist. One major cause of chronic daily headache is medication overuse. Patients may inadvertently overuse analgesics, triptans or ergotamine and convert an episodic headache syndrome into a chronic problem. Withdrawal of the overused medication may be achieved using transitional strategies to cover the period of withdrawal headache, e.g. with non-steroidal anti-inflammatory drugs (or steroids), antiemetics and dihydroergotamine. Preventive measures, notably tricyclic and related drugs, should be introduced at the earliest opportunity.

Facial pain

Many of the neurological syndromes described in this chapter may present with facial pain rather than headache (e.g., giant cell arteritis, cluster headache and migraine itself). There are, however, other distinctive syndromes where pain is restricted to the face.

Trigeminal neuralgia

This disorder, which typically affects patients older than 50 years, is attributable to compression of the trigeminal sensory root adjacent to the brainstem. It was previously subdivided into idiopathic and symptomatic cases. The latter include tumours of the cerebellopontine angle and, in younger patients, multiple sclerosis (where demyelination has affected the trigeminal sensory fibres within the brainstem). It is now clear that even in cases previously labelled idiopathic there is an identifiable cause of compression of the trigeminal sensory root, usually an aberrant arterial loop.

Patients present with unilateral facial pain within the distribution of one or more divisions of the trigeminal nerve (the mandibular and maxillary divisions being most commonly affected). The pain is **lancinating** in quality – brief, severe, sharp, stabbing, electric shock-like jolts of pain – though eventually a continuous background pain may also be present. There are often '**trigger**' areas, where even gentle pressure may produce pain. Thus, patients may be reluctant to wash their faces or shave, for fear of provoking an attack. Sometimes speaking or even a cold breeze is sufficient to produce pain. Chewing food may be difficult, with resultant weight loss. **Glossopharyngeal neuralgia** is a similar (rarer) disorder with pain in the throat or deep inside the ear. In general, patients with trigeminal neuralgia have normal trigeminal nerve function on examination. Anxiety about trigger areas may lead to involuntary facial spasms – '**tic douloureux**'. The presence of abnormal neurological signs increases the likelihood of an underlying lesion, e.g. tumour at the cerebellopontine angle, which may be identified by MR imaging.

Simple analgesics are generally of no use in trigeminal neuralgia. Most patients will, however, respond to **carbamazepine**, with adequate pain control. If carbamazepine is not tolerated or fails, other medical management, e.g. with baclofen, phenytoin, sodium valproate, gabapentin, clonazepam or tricyclic antidepressants, may be tried but is less likely to help. Surgical treatment may then be required. Previous operations, where the trigeminal ganglion was sectioned, often led to the unfortunate situation where the patient's pain persisted despite facial numbness – '**anaesthesia dolorosa**'. More selective procedures, e.g. glycerol injection into the ganglion or radiofrequency thermocoagulation, may be beneficial. Alternatively, the patient may require definitive posterior fossa exploration and decompression of the trigeminal sensory root.

Post-herpetic neuralgia

Patients who have suffered shingles in one of the branches of the trigeminal nerve (often the first – **zoster ophthalmicus**) may experience persistent facial pain after the rash has healed. The pain may be very severe and intractable, lasting 2–3 years after the eruption, but sometimes responds to tricyclic antidepressants, carbamazepine or topical application of capsaicin.

Atypical facial pain

Some patients present with constant facial pain in a non-anatomical distribution, and for which no local cause is found. Treatment is unsatisfactory but coexistent anxiety and/or depression may indicate potential benefit from tricyclic and related drugs, e.g. dosulepin.

Other causes of headache and facial pain

The neurological syndromes described in this chapter must be differentiated from local causes of pain, e.g. disease of the eyes, ears, nose and paranasal sinuses, throat or teeth. The site of the pain may be useful in the differential diagnosis (Fig. 9.1).

Miscellaneous causes of headache include pain triggered by coughing, exertion and sexual intercourse. Cough and exertional headaches are usually benign, but in some patients MR imaging reveals cerebellar tissue protruding into the foramen magnum (cerebellar ectopia). Coital headache is also usually benign but in some cases is severe and sudden enough to warrant investigation to exclude subarachnoid haemorrhage. 'Ice-pick' headaches are brief, sharp jabs of pain felt anywhere in the head, again generally benign.

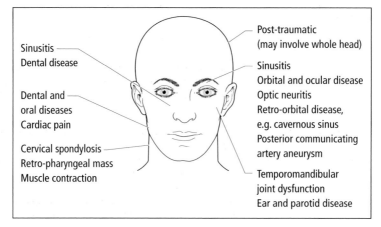

Figure 9.1 Local causes of headache and facial pain.

Sinusitis
Dental disease

Dental and
oral diseases
Cardiac pain

Cervical spondylosis
Retro-pharyngeal mass
Muscle contraction

Post-traumatic
(may involve whole head)

Sinusitis
Orbital and ocular disease
Optic neuritis
Retro-orbital disease,
e.g. cavernous sinus
Posterior communicating
artery aneurysm

Temporomandibular
joint dysfunction
Ear and parotid disease

Key points

- Headache may (rarely) signify a defined underlying pathophysiological process, e.g. raised intracranial pressure, meningeal irritation or giant cell arteritis
- Migraine may or may not be associated with an aura
- Migraine aura may mimic a transient ischaemic attack or epilepsy
- Migraine attacks may be treated acutely or prophylactically
- Trigeminal neuralgia is characterized by unilateral lancinating facial pain, typically provoked by specific 'triggers', and relieved by carbamazepine

Migraine

Case history: A 23-year-old woman presented with a 5-year history of episodic headache. Each attack began with her seeing 'black and white spots' in the left visual field. After 15–30 minutes, she would have blurred vision, affecting the entire left half-field. The visual disturbance then cleared and was followed by a severe throbbing headache always in the right occipital region, lasting up to 24 hours and associated with photophobia and vomiting. Initially, she had only two or three attacks per year, but for the 9 months leading to her presentation the frequency had deteriorated to at least two episodes per month. This worsening coincided with her having started the combined oral contraceptive. She had no other past history of note. In the family history, her mother had suffered from episodic headaches. There were no abnormalities on neurological or general examination.

Comment: The diagnosis of migraine is supported in this patient's case by the unilaterality and periodicity of the headaches; the visual aura, photophobia and vomiting; the quality and duration of the pain; and the positive family history. The fact that her headaches were *always* right-sided is not unusual in migraine – up to 20% of patients have attacks which are strictly 'side-locked'. However, given that she had such a stereotyped contralateral visual aura, she would certainly be investigated by MRI brain scan, looking in particular for an underlying vascular malformation in the right occipital lobe. A deterioration in the frequency of her migraines is predictable following the introduction of the combined oral contraceptive, which should be regarded as contraindicated in patients who have migraine with regular stereotyped aura.

Giant cell arteritis

Case history: A 66-year-old man presented with a 5-week history of bitemporal headache. He had noticed scalp tenderness when combing his hair. Over a similar period he had felt generally unwell with night sweats, anorexia and weight loss of 3 kg. There was pain and stiffness in his shoulders and hips in the mornings, and pain in his jaw when he chewed his food. Three days before presentation, he experienced transient loss of vision in the left eye, lasting 30 min. Examination confirmed scalp tenderness. Temporal artery pulsation was not palpable. The left optic disc appeared mildly swollen on fundoscopy.

Comment: This patient's history and examination are highly suggestive of a diagnosis of giant cell arteritis – subacute headache with scalp tenderness, constitutional symptoms and girdle pain, intermittent claudication of the jaw and ultimately an episode of amaurosis fugax. Transient monocular visual loss in giant cell arteritis is often of longer duration than that due to carotid embolism (Chapter 11). Once the diagnosis is suspected, treatment is urgent to prevent permanent loss of vision. The correct management of this patient is to take blood immediately for ESR (and full blood count, C-reactive protein (CRP), glucose and liver function), and give 200 mg intravenous hydrocortisone without delay, followed by prednisolone 60 mg daily. A temporal artery biopsy should then be done at the earliest opportunity. A positive histological result is very helpful in the management of a patient who is likely to remain on steroids for 2 years or more. A negative result would not necessarily dissuade the clinician from continuing treatment, but in such circumstances there would be increased reliance on the clinical response to treatment and on further investigation to exclude alternative causes. Occasionally the ESR is normal in giant cell arteritis, but CRP is almost always elevated.

See also Subarachnoid haemorrhage (Chapter 11), Headache due to intracranial tumour (Chapter 13).

Chapter 10

Epilepsy

Definitions

The physiological definition of epilepsy is un-changed from that provided by Hughlings Jackson in the nineteenth century:

Epilepsy is the name for occasional, sudden, ex-cessive, rapid and local discharges of grey matter.

Clinically, epilepsy is a paroxysmal disorder in which cerebral cortical neuronal discharges result in intermittent, stereotyped attacks of altered con-sciousness, motor or sensory function, behaviour or emotion.

A distinction must be drawn between an iso-lated seizure and the recurring tendency to seizures which is epilepsy.

Classification and causes

Epileptic seizures are broadly classified by whether their onset is focal (**partial**) or **generalized**. Par-tial seizures are further subclassifed as:
- **Simple partial seizures**, where consciousness is retained throughout the attack;
- **Complex partial seizures**, where conscious-ness is impaired at any stage.

Lecture Notes: Neurology, 9th edition. By Lionel Ginsberg. Published 2010 by Blackwell Publishing.

Partial seizures may become **secondarily generalized**, the patient losing conscious-ness with clinical evidence of spread across the cerebral cortex, e.g. bilateral convulsive movements.

A more detailed classification of epilepsy within these broad categories, according to clinical and EEG characteristics, is given in Table 10.1.

Epilepsy may also be subdivided according to whether it is **idiopathic** (most patients) or **symp-tomatic**, i.e. where a cause can be found. Causes of symptomatic epilepsy are listed in Table 10.2. Idiopathic epilepsy frequently shows a strong in-herited predisposition.

Epidemiology

Up to 1% of the general population suffer from active epilepsy, with 20–50 new patients being di-agnosed per 100,000 per year. The approximate annual death rate for epilepsy is 2 per 100,000. Deaths may relate directly to seizures, for example when there is an uncontrolled series of seizures, the patient failing to regain consciousness be-tween attacks (**status epilepticus** – Chapter 20), or when accidental injury has occurred. The phe-nomenon of sudden unexplained death in peo-ple with epilepsy is usually assumed to be related to seizure activity and possibly to associated car-diorespiratory dysfunction.

Table 10.1 Classification of epilepsy.

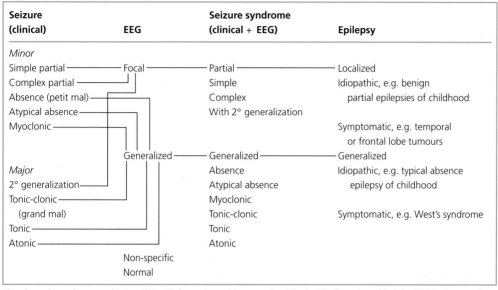

Seizure (clinical)	EEG	Seizure syndrome (clinical + EEG)	Epilepsy
Minor			
Simple partial ——————— Focal ———————		Partial ———————	Localized
Complex partial ———————		Simple	Idiopathic, e.g. benign
Absence (petit mal) ———————		Complex	partial epilepsies of childhood
Atypical absence ———————		With 2° generalization	
Myoclonic ———————			Symptomatic, e.g. temporal
			or frontal lobe tumours
	Generalized ———————	Generalized ———————	Generalized
Major		Absence	Idiopathic, e.g. typical absence
2° generalization ———————		Atypical absence	epilepsy of childhood
Tonic-clonic ———————		Myoclonic	
(grand mal)		Tonic-clonic	Symptomatic, e.g. West's syndrome
Tonic ———————		Tonic	
Atonic ———————		Atonic	
	Non-specific		
	Normal		

This chart shows how combining clinical information with neurophysiological findings (provided the EEG is abnormal) helps subclassify minor and major seizures. The individual seizure types and syndromes are described in more detail in the text.

Important epileptic syndromes: adulthood

Primary generalized epilepsy

Although often beginning in childhood, primary generalized epilepsy in adults presents a common management problem and the most typical seizure type (**tonic-clonic** or **grand mal**) is so distinctive as to warrant separate description.

Before an attack, patients may experience vague symptoms of dizziness or irritability. The convulsion itself may begin with an **epileptic cry**. The patient loses consciousness and falls to the ground. During the first, or **tonic** phase, generalized muscle spasms occur, lasting only a few seconds. In the subsequent **clonic** phase, there are sharp repetitive muscular jerks. Tongue biting, incontinence of urine and salivation may occur. When the jerking stops, patients usually remain unconscious for approximately 30 minutes and afterwards are confused and drowsy for several hours. On recovery, there is usually a headache and stiffness or injury from the fall. Back pain is common; indeed, mus-

cular spasms may be of sufficient violence to result in vertebral fractures. This type of epilepsy is usually controllable with one drug.

Partial epilepsy

Temporal lobe epilepsy

In these seizures, an aura or warning of the attack may consist of psychic symptoms (e.g., fear or a sensation of **déjà vu**), hallucinations (olfactory, gustatory or formed visual images) or simply a rising sensation in the epigastrium. Patients may become confused and anxious, and exhibit organized, stereotyped movements (**automatism**). These include chewing and lip smacking, but may be more complex and sometimes aggressive and violent.

Jacksonian epilepsy

These focal motor attacks typically begin in the corner of the mouth, the thumb and index finger or the great toe. Movements rapidly spread across

Table 10.2 Causes of symptomatic epilepsy.

Neonates
Birth trauma
Intracranial haemorrhage
Hypoxia
Hypoglycaemia
Hypocalcaemia

Children
Congenital anomalies
Tuberous sclerosis (Chapter 18)
Metabolic storage diseases

Young adults
Head injuries
Drugs and alcohol

Middle-aged adults
Cerebral tumour

Elderly
Cerebrovascular disease
Degenerative disorders (Alzheimer's, prion diseases)

Not all the above causes are strictly age-specific; e.g.
    tumours may present at other ages

Some causes are not restricted to individual age groups:
    Infection, e.g. meningitis, encephalitis, abscess,
        cysticercosis
    Inflammation – multiple sclerosis (rarely), vasculitis
    Metabolic encephalopathy (Chapter 19)

the face or ascend the limb (**Jacksonian march**). Jacksonian epilepsy is generally associated with underlying organic brain disease, e.g. tumour in the region of the motor cortex. After such an attack, the affected limb(s) may remain temporarily weak (**Todd's paralysis**).

Epilepsia partialis continua is a rare form of Jacksonian epilepsy, where the attack persists for days, weeks or even months.

Important epileptic syndromes: childhood and adolescence

This section deals only with syndromes that may have consequences in adulthood.

Febrile convulsions

Seizures associated with fever:
• occur in 3% of otherwise normal children aged 3 months to 5 years,

• are usually brief (less than 15 minutes) and generalized, though some children have focal, prolonged attacks, sometimes with residual neurological signs,
• occur as an isolated attack without recurrence in 70% of cases,
• carry a risk of subsequent epilepsy in 2–5% of cases,
• generally do not require treatment with prophylactic anti-epilepsy drugs.

Infantile spasms (West's syndrome)

These consist of a triad of:
• brief spasms beginning within the first few months of life, characteristically shock-like flexion of arms, head and neck with drawing up of the knees (**salaam attack**),
• progressive learning difficulties,
• characteristic EEG abnormality (**hypsarrhythmia**).

In a minority of patients the condition is idiopathic but usually a cause can be identified, e.g. perinatal asphyxia, encephalitis, metabolic disorders and cerebral malformations.

Most conventional anticonvulsant drugs are ineffective (though sodium valproate and vigabatrin may be beneficial). The treatment of choice is often with corticosteroids.

Absence epilepsy ('petit mal')

• This condition typically starts in childhood (peak age of onset 4–8 years, commoner in girls), though there is also a juvenile form.
• The attacks (typical absences) occur without warning. The child stares blankly into space and stops talking. The eyes may flutter or roll up under the lids. Recovery occurs within seconds and there may be many attacks daily.
• Absences are associated with characteristic EEG abnormalities: 3-Hz generalized, symmetrical spike–wave complexes (Fig. 10.1).
• Treatment is with sodium valproate, ethosuximide or both.

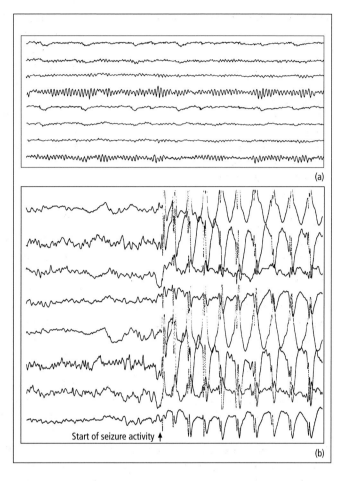

Figure 10.1 EEG tracings. (a) Normal and (b) typical childhood absence epilepsy (petit mal).

Start of seizure activity ↑

(a)

(b)

• Patients may subsequently develop other seizure types – the overall risk of seizures as an adult following childhood absence epilepsy is approximately 10%.

Juvenile myoclonic epilepsy (Janz syndrome)

This is increasingly recognized as a common form of primary generalized epilepsy; age of onset is typically in the teens.

Patients have the clinical triad of:
• infrequent generalized seizures, often on waking,
• daytime absences,
• sudden, shock-like, involuntary jerking movements (**myoclonus**), usually in the morning. Patients may, therefore, apparently inexplicably spill their breakfast or throw it across the room ('Kellogg's epilepsy').

The EEG shows polyspike–wave discharges and photosensitivity. Treatment with sodium valproate is often successful, but recurrence is likely if medication is stopped. Alternative drugs include clonazepam, levetiracetam and lamotrigine. This benign condition must be distinguished from childhood conditions where severe myoclonus and epilepsy are associated with underlying degenerative disease of the brain (progressive

Table 10.3 Differential diagnosis of epilepsy.

Syncope
Cardiac dysrhythmia
Pseudoseizures
Hyperventilation/panic attacks
Transient ischaemic attacks
Migraine
Narcolepsy
Hypoglycaemia
Vestibular disorders

myoclonic epilepsies). Recognition of juvenile myoclonic epilepsy is important, as patients treated incorrectly with carbamazepine, rather than valproate, may worsen.

Investigation and diagnosis

The diagnosis of epilepsy is primarily clinical, based on a description of the seizures, usually from a witness as the patient may be unaware of any symptoms. The differential diagnosis is summarized in Table 10.3. Of these, the most important differentials are syncope (Chapter 2) and **pseudoseizures** (Chapter 19, simulated attacks, either unconsciously – 'hysterical' fits, or consciously – malingering).

Investigation of a patient with suspected epilepsy has the following aims:

- confirming or supporting the clinical diagnosis,
- classifying the epileptic syndrome,
- establishing a cause.

The EEG has a role in the first two aims, particularly in children. However, in adults there are frequent false-positive and false-negative recordings. Thus, minor non-specific EEG abnormalities may be detected in the normal population, and many patients with epilepsy show no abnormalities on repeated recordings between attacks (inter-ictal EEG). The yield of EEG can be increased by prolonged recordings, particularly after sleep deprivation. In some patients, ultimate proof of the diagnosis of epilepsy is obtained only by ambulatory EEG or **telemetry** with simultaneous video recording of symptomatic events.

Routine blood tests, e.g. serum glucose and calcium, have a role in achieving the third aim of investigating a patient with epilepsy, i.e. establishing the cause. Of far greater importance is brain imaging, by CT or MR scanning. This is particularly indicated in epilepsy of later onset, presenting as partial attacks, with or without focal neurological signs and EEG abnormalities. However, adult patients presenting with an isolated seizure will nowadays generally expect a brain scan, despite the low yield and limited influence on management of scan findings in such an unselected population.

Management

Drug treatment

Most neurologists will not prescribe prophylactic anti-epilepsy drugs after a single isolated seizure, but will introduce drug treatment after a second attack. The choice of drug is determined by the type of epileptic syndrome (Table 10.4). In

Table 10.4 Anti-epilepsy drugs and epileptic syndromes.

Seizure type	Drugs of choice
Partial	Carbamazepine
	Sodium valproate
	Phenytoin
	Lamotrigine
Absence	Ethosuximide
	Sodium valproate
	Lamotrigine
Myoclonic	Sodium valproate
	Clonazepam
	Lamotrigine
Generalized tonic-clonic	Sodium valproate
	Phenytoin
	Carbamazepine
	Lamotrigine

Other anti-epilepsy drugs have an important role as add-on therapy, particularly for partial seizures resistant to first-line drugs alone. Some of the newer drugs are also beginning to be used as monotherapy.

general, careful outpatient follow-up is required to establish the minimum effective dosage and monitor for side effects. Measurement of blood levels of anti-epilepsy drugs may be helpful. Most patients' epilepsy (70%) will be adequately controlled with a single drug (**monotherapy**). A further group will require the addition of a second drug. When patients are on three or more drugs, the likelihood of completely successful medical treatment is low. Reasons for refractory epilepsy include:

- non-concordance with medication,
- pseudoseizures or non-epileptic attacks (either alone or in combination with genuine seizures),
- associated structural brain disease, e.g. developmental anomalies, which may or may not be amenable to surgery (see below),
- alcohol and lifestyle.

Disregarding the small group of patients with refractory epilepsy, the long-term prognosis of epilepsy is good, most patients attaining a 5-year remission and many successfully stopping treatment. The decision to stop treatment in an adult will be determined by:

- duration of remission,
- type of epilepsy,
- effect of seizure recurrence on driving and employment (see below),
- side effects of treatment.

Specific management problems of epilepsy in pregnancy and of status epilepticus are discussed in Chapters 19 and 20, respectively.

Important pharmacological aspects of the major anti-epilepsy drugs are summarized in Table 10.5. Drugs with more limited indications, or of more recent availability, are listed in Table 10.6.

Surgical treatment

Patients with intractable epilepsy, refractory to optimal doses of anti-epilepsy drugs, are increasingly being considered for neurosurgical procedures. There is particular interest in patients who have a definable site of seizure onset. Small temporal lobe lesions, sclerotic or developmental (hamartomatous) in origin, previously missed on CT scan, are now detectable by more sophisticated MR imaging techniques as shown in Fig. 10.2. In other patients, where no lesion is found on imaging, an epileptogenic focus may be localized electrophysiologically. These patients may then undergo selective removal of the epileptogenic tissue. In others, less specific symptomatic surgical procedures may be indicated, including hemispherectomy and disconnection procedures, e.g. section of the corpus callosum. In all cases, surgical treatment is reserved for use only in carefully selected patients, assessed in neuroscience centres, including determination of the functional importance of any tissue to be removed.

Other aspects

Specific triggers for epileptic seizures are only infrequently recognized, but patients should avoid alcohol and some may have attacks provoked by flickering lights, e.g. television and computer screens. Other forms of treatment for epilepsy including dietary (e.g., ketogenic diet) are of unproven benefit. The psychological consequences of a diagnosis of epilepsy are still often underestimated but may include depression and personality disorder. Social aspects include the following.

Epilepsy and driving

In general, in the UK, people with a history of epilepsy may drive only after a seizure-free interval of at least 6 months, and should inform the Driver and Vehicle Licensing Agency. More stringent restrictions apply to drivers of heavy goods and passenger-carrying vehicles. Sleep-related epilepsy is a special situation. Patients may drive if they have an established pattern of seizures occurring only in relation to sleep during the previous 3 years.

Table 10.5 Major anti-epilepsy drugs.

Drug	Mode of action	Pharmacokinetics	Side effects	
			Dose-related	Allergic
Carbamazepine	'Membrane stabilizer' Limits repetitive firing of action potentials	Initial low dosage Controlled-release preparation permits twice-daily regime Blood levels limited value	Giddiness Nausea Drowsiness	Rashes Leucopenia
Sodium valproate	Uncertain – multiple	Controlled-release preparation permits twice-or even once-daily regime Blood levels little value	Tremor Confusion Chronic toxicity: alopecia, weight gain	Hepatitis
Phenytoin	'Membrane stabilizer'	Once-daily regime Narrow therapeutic range Blood levels useful	Drowsiness Ataxia Chronic toxicity: gum hypertrophy, acne, hirsutism, coarsening of facial features, folate deficiency	Rashes Lymphadenopathy
Lamotrigine	'Membrane stabilizer'	Half-life prolonged by sodium valproate Dosing schedule depends on concomitant drug treatment	Nausea Dizziness Tremor Headache	Rash Fever Arthralgia Lymphadenopathy Eosinophilia Stevens–Johnson syndrome

Employment

There are statutory barriers to the employment of epileptic patients in certain occupations, particularly the armed services and emergency services, and as aircraft pilots and train drivers.

Leisure activities

Swimming and rock and tree climbing should be restricted to situations where there is adequate supervision.

Table 10.6 Other anti-epilepsy drugs.

Older anti-epilepsy drugs retaining specific uses:

Phenobarbitone (and primidone)

Many patients with long-standing epilepsy remain on these drugs

Primidone is metabolized to phenobarbitone

Withdrawal seizures are likely if phenobarbitone is stopped abruptly

Phenobarbitone retains a role in the management of status epilepticus (Chapter 20)

Ethosuximide

Used in childhood absence epilepsy (petit mal)

May exacerbate tonic-clonic seizures

Clonazepam

Effective in myoclonic and absence epilepsy

May be administered intravenously in status epilepticus

Clobazam

Add-on therapy in tonic-clonic and partial seizures, especially if perimenstrual

Newer drugs used predominantly as add-on therapy for partial seizures:

Vigabatrin

Also used as monotherapy for infantile spasms (West's syndrome)

Avoid in patients with a psychiatric history

Associated with irreversible peripheral visual field defects in about one-third of patients

For this reason nowadays only used in exceptional circumstances outside the context of West's syndrome

Gabapentin

Also used in the management of neurogenic pain

Unlike many other anti-epilepsy drugs is eliminated by the renal route rather than hepatic metabolism

Topiramate

Also used as adjunctive treatment for primary generalized tonic-clonic seizures

Avoid in patients with a history of renal stones

Tiagabine

Oxcarbazepine

Similar indications to carbamazepine, probably has a better side effect profile

Levetiracetam

Increasingly used as monotherapy

May cause behavioural and mood change

Pregabalin

Useful in patients with epilepsy and generalized anxiety disorder

Zonisamide

Risk of renal calculi

Lacosamide

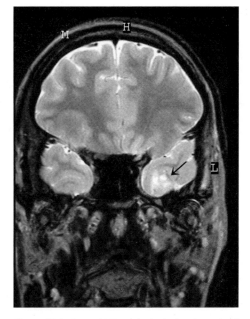

Figure 10.2 Coronal MRI of the brain showing a developmental abnormality of the temporal lobe (arrowed), which acted as an epileptogenic focus.

Key points

- In epilepsy, paroxysmal cerebral cortical discharges lead to stereotyped attacks, typically affecting consciousness, behaviour, emotion, motor or sensory function
- Seizures may be partial or generalized; epilepsy may be idiopathic or symptomatic
- The differential diagnosis of epilepsy includes syncope and pseudoseizures
- Anti-epilepsy drug treatment is generally reserved until a patient experiences a second epileptic seizure
- Most patients achieve good seizure control with a single drug (monotherapy)
- A small minority of selected patients with refractory epilepsy may benefit from neurosurgical intervention
- A seizure-free interval of 6 months is generally required in the UK before patients can resume driving

Juvenile myoclonic epilepsy

Case history: A 16-year-old female patient suffered a generalized convulsion with tongue biting. For 6 months previously she had been experiencing jerking of her upper limbs in the morning, often spilling her coffee at breakfast. Her general practitioner prescribed carbamazepine but, if anything, the jerking worsened. She had no other past history of note. In the family history, a cousin had epilepsy. Neurological examination was normal.

Comment: The diagnosis of juvenile myoclonic epilepsy rests on the clinical triad of generalized convulsions (usually infrequent), morning myoclonus and daytime absences. There is often a family history. This patient had no history of absences but the combination of an isolated seizure and morning myoclonus was highly suggestive of the diagnosis, and 'formes frustes' are recognised. The condition is usually very sensitive to treatment with sodium valproate, but doctors are naturally reluctant to use this as a first-line anti-epilepsy drug in women of childbearing age because of the risk of teratogenicity and its other side effects. Carbamazepine may, in fact, worsen symptoms, and other drugs, e.g. clonazepam, lamotrigine and levetiracetam, may not be as effective as sodium valproate. Though the onset of juvenile myoclonic epilepsy is usually in the teens, 'juvenile' is a misnomer in the sense that treatment is lifelong, with a high risk of recurrent symptoms on attempted anti-epilepsy drug withdrawal.

Complex partial seizures of temporal lobe origin

Case history: A 23-year-old woman had suffered several febrile convulsions in infancy. From the age of 11 years, she had seizures which were preceded by a feeling of faintness and palpitations. A generalized convulsion with tongue biting would follow. These were not controlled by phenobarbitone or phenytoin, but there was an improvement when her medication was changed to carbamazepine. On this drug, she had no further generalized convulsions but experienced three or four episodes per month, where she described herself as 'going vacant' for a few seconds. None of these had been witnessed. There was no other past history and no family history of epilepsy. Neurological examination was normal.

Comment: Though the features were rather non-specific, there was sufficient history to suggest that this patient's convulsions were preceded by an aura and that they were therefore due to secondary generalization. Her initial treatment had been in a country with limited availability of anti-epilepsy drugs, hence the use of drugs which would not be considered first line in developed countries. Despite some improvement with carbamazepine, she continued to experience quite frequent complex partial seizures and was investigated. A MRI brain scan showed right-sided hippocampal sclerosis, for which her history of febrile convulsions in infancy is a risk factor. EEG confirmed an epileptogenic focus in the right temporal lobe. Other anti-epilepsy drug combinations were unsuccessful and she was referred for consideration of epilepsy surgery.

Chapter 11

Stroke

Definitions

Stroke is a syndrome consisting of rapidly developing (usually seconds or minutes) symptoms and/or signs of loss of focal (or sometimes global) CNS function. The symptoms last more than 24 hours or lead to death.

Vascular mechanisms causing stroke may be classified as:
- infarction (embolic or thrombotic),
- haemorrhage.

A **transient ischaemic attack** is a rapid loss of focal CNS (including retinal) function, lasting less than 24 hours, and presumed caused by embolic, thrombotic or haemodynamic vascular mechanisms. Some transient episodes last longer than 24 hours, yet patients recover completely – **reversible ischaemic neurological deficits**.

Epidemiology

Stroke is the third most common cause of death in developed countries, after heart disease and cancer. The annual incidence is 2 per 1000 population. The majority of strokes are cerebral infarcts.

Lecture Notes: Neurology, 9th edition. By Lionel Ginsberg. Published 2010 by Blackwell Publishing.

Infarction in the CNS

Aetiology and pathogenesis

Thrombosis of arteries (or veins) in the CNS may be attributable to one or more of **Virchow's triad**:
- abnormalities of the vessel wall, commonly degenerative disease but also inflammation (**vasculitis**) or trauma (**dissection**),
- abnormalities of the blood, e.g. polycythaemia,
- disturbances of blood flow.

Embolism may complicate degenerative disease of the arteries to the CNS, or it may arise from the heart:
- valvular disease,
- atrial fibrillation,
- recent myocardial infarction.

The most common cause of stroke is degenerative arterial disease, either **atherosclerosis** in larger vessels (with consequent thromboembolism) or small vessel disease (**lipohyalinosis**). The probability of developing significant degenerative arterial disease is increased by certain **vascular risk factors** (Table 11.1).

Pathophysiology

When an artery is acutely occluded by thrombus or embolus, the area of the CNS supplied by it will undergo infarction if there is no adequate

Table 11.1 Vascular risk factors.

Age
Family history of vascular disease
Hypertension
Diabetes mellitus
Smoking
Hypercholesterolaemia
Alcohol
Oral contraceptives
Plasma fibrinogen

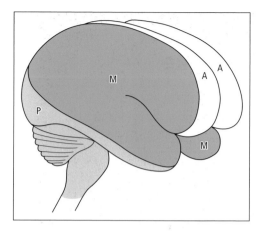

Figure 11.1 The distribution of the anterior (A), middle (M) and posterior (P) cerebral arteries. The anterior (carotid) circulation consists of A + M, the posterior circulation is P plus the branches supplying the brainstem and cerebellum.

collateral blood supply. Surrounding a central necrotic zone, an **'ischaemic penumbra'** remains viable for a time, i.e. it may recover function if blood flow is restored.

CNS ischaemia may be accompanied by **swelling** for two reasons:

• **cytotoxic oedema** – accumulation of water in damaged glial cells and neurones,

• **vasogenic oedema** – extracellular fluid accumulation as a result of breakdown of the **blood–brain barrier**.

In the brain, this swelling may be sufficient to produce clinical deterioration in the days following a major stroke, as a result of a rise in intracranial pressure and compression of adjacent structures.

Clinical features and classification

Symptoms and signs of arterial infarcts depend on the vascular territory affected (Fig. 11.1).

• Total anterior (carotid) circulation infarct
  • hemiplegia (damage to the upper part of the corticospinal tract),
  • hemianopia (damage to the optic radiation),
  • cortical deficits, e.g. dysphasia (dominant hemisphere), visuo-spatial loss (non-dominant hemisphere).

• Partial anterior circulation infarct
  • two of the above, or cortical deficit alone.

• Lacunar infarct
  • intrinsic disease (lipohyalinosis) in a small deep (perforating) artery producing a characteristic syndrome, e.g. pure motor or sensory stroke, or ataxic hemiparesis. Multiple lacunar infarcts may produce cumulative neurological deficits, including cognitive impairment (**multi-infarct dementia**) and a gait disorder characterized by small steps (marche à petits pas) and difficulty starting walking (ignition failure) – **'gait apraxia'**.

• Posterior (vertebrobasilar) circulation infarct
  • evidence of brainstem lesion (e.g., vertigo, diplopia, altered consciousness),
  • homonymous hemianopia.

• Spinal cord infarction, Chapter 15.

Investigations and diagnosis

Stroke is a clinical diagnosis. Investigations are directed towards:

• establishing the cause,

• preventing recurrence and, in severely affected patients, identifying factors that may lead to further deterioration in CNS function.

Common investigations in patients with stroke therefore include:

• full blood count and ESR,

• urea, electrolytes, glucose and lipids,

• chest radiograph and ECG,

• CT cranial scan (Fig. 11.2).

CT scanning is useful for distinguishing between cerebral infarction and haemorrhage, which may

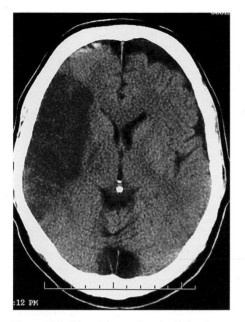

:12 PM

Figure 11.2 CT cranial scan of cerebral infarction.

influence early management. It also eliminates important differential diagnoses (intracranial tumour, subdural haematoma).

Complications and course

Severely affected patients, e.g. immobilized with dense hemiplegia, are prone to complications that may lead to early death, including:
- pneumonia (over 50% of stroke patients are acutely dysphagic, with a risk of aspiration, though swallowing recovers spontaneously in most patients), septicaemia (via pressure sores or urinary tract infection),
- deep vein thrombosis and pulmonary embolism,
- myocardial infarction, arrhythmias and heart failure,
- fluid imbalance.

Approximately 10% of patients with cerebral infarction die in the first 30 days. Up to 50% of survivors remain dependent. Factors contributing to long-term disability include:
- pressure sores,
- epilepsy,
- recurrent falls and fractures,
- spasticity, with pain, contractures and frozen shoulder,
- depression.

Treatment

The acute management of ischaemic stroke comprises:
- Admission to a **stroke unit** (Chapter 21),
- Aspirin 300 mg daily, modest benefit when given within 48 hours of onset,
- **Thrombolysis.** Up to 15% of patients will be eligible for thrombolysis with intravenous tissue plasminogen activator (alteplase). Patient assessment is urgent because this drug treatment must be started within 3 hours of stroke onset. Though the time window may be extended to 4.5 hours, or beyond, treatment should be as early as possible to minimize permanent brain injury. The key steps in a thrombolysis protocol are rapid transfer to hospital and equally rapid clinical assessment including CT brain scan to exclude intracranial haemorrhage. Patients are ineligible for thrombolysis if there is uncertainty about the exact time of stroke onset and if they have risk factors for intracranial or systemic haemorrhage. For eligible patients, the benefits of preventing death or dependency outweigh the risk of alteplase causing symptomatic intracerebral haemorrhage. Some patients may benefit from newer techniques such as intra-arterial thrombolysis and clot retrieval, but these have not been the subjects of controlled clinical trials.
- Surgery is rarely needed in acute stroke management. Some patients with cerebellar infarction may require urgent posterior fossa decompression and ventricular drainage if swelling caused by the infarct is leading to brainstem compression and obstruction to CSF flow. Young patients with total middle cerebral artery infarction may develop massive cerebral oedema with a high risk of raised intracranial pressure, brainstem compression and death ("malignant MCA occlusion syndrome"). Temporary removal of the skull vault on the side of the infarct (hemicraniectomy) may be life-saving.

Prevention

Recurrence may be prevented by modifying risk factors, especially stopping smoking and, to a lesser extent, manipulating diet (low animal fat, low salt, avoiding excess alcohol) and prescribing cholesterol-lowering agents, i.e. statins. In the long term, control of blood pressure is also important. For the first 2 weeks after an ischaemic stroke, however, patients should not receive antihypertensive therapy beyond their pre-existing treatment unless there is evidence of malignant hypertension. This is because too rapid lowering of blood pressure may worsen ischaemia in a region where the cerebral circulation is already compromised (see below).

Lifelong antiplatelet treatment is indicated, commencing as soon as possible after a cerebral infarct. The initial dose of aspirin (300 mg daily) can be reduced to 75 mg daily after 4 weeks. Anticoagulation with warfarin is effective prophylaxis in the presence of atrial fibrillation and other cardiac sources of embolism.

Rehabilitation

Early management in stroke units is potentially life-saving (Chapter 21). Such an environment is best suited to the meticulous control of important variables which can affect outcome, e.g. hydration, temperature and blood glucose, along with appropriate management for swallowing difficulties and to prevent venous thromboembolism. Subsequent continued physiotherapy, occupational and speech therapy, and the involvement of social services may help survivors regain independence.

Hypotension and hypertension

Cerebral blood flow is normally maintained at a relatively constant level through a range of blood pressure (typically 80–180 mm Hg systolic) by **autoregulation** (Fig. 11.3). In this process, intracerebral arteries alter their calibre in response to changes in cerebral perfusion pressure (the difference between blood pressure and intracranial pressure), a fall in pressure producing a widening of vessel lumen and hence constant flow.

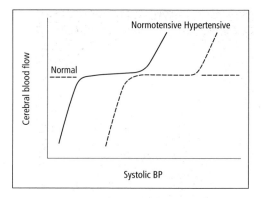

Figure 11.3 Cerebral autoregulation in normotensive and hypertensive individuals.

If blood pressure falls below the autoregulatory range, as may occur in hypovolaemic shock, cerebral infarction may result as blood vessels are unable to dilate further in response to the drop in pressure, and blood flow falls. The regions most likely to be affected are the **border zones** or **watersheds** between vascular territories, as perfusion pressure here is usually at its lowest. Thus, for example, the patient may develop visual field defects or more complex visual disturbances (e.g., visual agnosia) as a result of infarction at the border zone between posterior and middle cerebral artery territories.

With severe (malignant) hypertension, the autoregulatory range may be exceeded and cerebral blood flow rises, with damage to vessel walls (**fibrinoid necrosis**) and consequent cerebral oedema. Patients develop features of raised intracranial pressure – headache, vomiting, drowsiness and papilloedema – along with seizures and focal neurological signs.

Treatment of **hypertensive encephalopathy** is by prompt lowering of the blood pressure, aiming at a diastolic pressure of 100–110 mm Hg initially (more drastic lowering may result in cerebral infarction if long-standing hypertension has shifted the autoregulatory curve to the right).

Venous infarction

Thrombosis of the intracranial venous sinuses produces clinical syndromes distinct from arterial

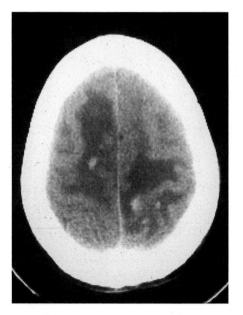

Figure 11.4 Superior sagittal sinus thrombosis. CT cranial scan showing low-density areas of ischaemia/infarction along with high-density haemorrhagic regions in both cerebral hemispheres.

infarction. Thus, **superior sagittal sinus thrombosis** (Fig. 11.4) may present with:

• headache, papilloedema and other features resembling benign (idiopathic) intracranial hypertension (Chapter 9),

• early seizures,

• bilateral signs of neurological deficit, often progressive, with impairment of consciousness.

It has many causes, including:

• the puerperium,

• dehydration,

• cachexia,

• coagulopathies,

• oral contraceptives.

Other venous sinuses affected by thrombosis include the cavernous sinus (producing a red swollen eyelid and conjunctiva, III, IV, VI, Va and Vb cranial nerve palsies and papilloedema) and the lateral sinus (raised intracranial pressure, seizures and drowsiness).

The latter two sinuses may undergo thrombosis as a result of spread of infection (from the face and

orbit to the cavernous sinus, and from the ear to the lateral sinus).

Treatment of intracranial venous sinus thrombosis is aimed at the underlying cause, in particular eradicating infection with appropriate antibiotics. Formal intravenous **heparinization** is beneficial in non-infective cases, but there may be concern about the use of anticoagulants in the presence of haemorrhagic venous infarction of the brain.

Transient ischaemic attacks

Aetiology

Transient ischaemic attacks (TIAs) are most commonly caused by thromboembolism from atheromatous neck vessels. Other causes are lipohyalinosis of intracranial small vessels and cardiogenic embolism. More rarely, they may be due to vasculitis or haematological disease.

Clinical features

The hallmark of a TIA is sudden loss of focal CNS function; symptoms such as syncope, confusion and dizziness are therefore insufficient for the diagnosis. TIAs typically last minutes, not hours. The arterial territory of the attack will determine the symptoms:

• **Carotid** (most common)
  • hemiparesis,
  • hemisensory loss,
  • dysphasia,
  • monocular visual loss (**amaurosis fugax**) caused by retinal ischaemia;
• Vertebrobasilar
  • bilateral or alternating paresis or sensory loss,
  • bilateral sudden visual loss (in older patients),
  • diplopia, ataxia, vertigo, dysphagia – at least two of these simultaneously.

Some symptoms do not localize accurately to a specific arterial territory, e.g. hemianopia or dysarthria alone, though these are usually taken to be vertebrobasilar.

Neurological signs are usually absent by the time the patient is seen by a doctor, but **cholesterol emboli** may be visible on ophthalmoscopy in

Table 11.2 Differential diagnosis of transient ischaemic attacks.

> Migraine with aura
> Partial epilepsy
> Intracranial tumour, vascular malformation or chronic
>   subdural haematoma
> Multiple sclerosis
> Vestibular disorders
> Peripheral nerve or root lesions (e.g., radial nerve palsy)
> Hypoglycaemia
> Hyperventilation and other psychogenic processes

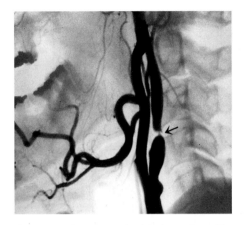

Figure 11.5 Severe stenosis of the internal carotid artery (arrowed).

patients with amaurosis fugax. A **carotid bruit** may be audible and is of particular relevance if on the appropriate side of a carotid TIA. Cardiac arrhythmias and murmurs may point to a cardiac source of embolism. A rare cause of vertebrobasilar TIAs is the **subclavian steal syndrome**. Here, stenosis of the proximal subclavian artery (sometimes with a bruit low in the neck and reduction in blood pressure and pulse volume in the ipsilateral arm) may lead to retrograde flow down the vertebral artery when the arm is exercised.

Investigations and diagnosis

The recognition of TIAs depends on the history. Their differential diagnosis is given in Table 11.2. Investigations are directed towards identifying the cause and hence preventing a more serious recurrence, i.e. stroke:
- full blood count, ESR,
- blood glucose and cholesterol,
- syphilis serology,
- ECG.
- chest radiograph, echocardiogram, 24-hour ECG – when cardiogenic embolism is suspected,
- CT cranial scan – to detect pre-existing cerebrovascular disease, also to exclude the remote possibility of a structural lesion, e.g. tumour, presenting with symptoms suggesting a TIA,
- carotid ultrasound or angiography – to detect carotid stenosis in patients with TIAs in carotid territory (Fig. 11.5),
- blood cultures – when infective endocarditis is suspected.

Prognosis and treatment

The risk of stroke in the first 5 years after a TIA is approximately 7% per annum, the greatest risk being in the first year, indeed the first hours, days and weeks. Coupled with an increased risk of myocardial infarction after TIA, the combined risk of stroke, myocardial infarct or vascular death is 9% per annum. Up to 15% of patients presenting with their first stroke will have had preceding TIAs. These facts underline the importance of identification of TIAs in the prevention of stroke. Patients' risk of stroke after TIA can be stratified, depending on whether they are older, diabetic or hypertensive, and on the description and duration of the event. High-risk patients should be assessed within 24 hours of an event, low-risk individuals within one week, so that preventive measures can be instituted as soon as possible. These measures include:
- modifying risk factors
  - treating hypertension,
  - stopping smoking,
  - reducing serum cholesterol by diet and drugs;
- antiplatelet drugs (low-dose aspirin):
  - contraindicated in active peptic ulcer disease,
  - some evidence suggests combined aspirin plus dipyridamole is more effective than either agent alone,
  - clopidogrel is an alternative antiplatelet drug for patients unable to tolerate aspirin;

- anticoagulants (warfarin)
  - when cardiogenic embolism has been identified, including non-rheumatic atrial fibrillation;
- carotid endarterectomy
  - surgical intervention to clear atheroma from
  the origin of the internal carotid artery is warranted for symptomatic severe carotid stenosis
  (greater than 70% stenosis), after TIAs or indeed
  minor stroke. Carotid angioplasty and stenting
  is a viable alternative to surgery.

The role of surgery for less severe or asymptomatic carotid stenoses is not so well established.
At present, there is no surgical option for most vertebrobasilar TIAs (with the rare exception of the
subclavian steal syndrome), though selected patients have been treated by vertebral angioplasty
and stenting.

Intracranial haemorrhage

Traumatic causes of intracranial haemorrhage are
discussed in Chapter 13.

Subarachnoid haemorrhage

Aetiology

Bleeding into the subarachnoid space is most commonly from:
- rupture of an aneurysm – congenital weaken-
ings occurring typically at junctions in the circle
of Willis (Fig. 11.6),

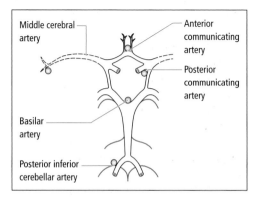

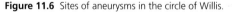

Figure 11.6 Sites of aneurysms in the circle of Willis.

- arteriovenous malformations (angiomas) –
anomalous malformed vessels, also congenital,
which enlarge and present in adult life.
   Rarer causes include:
- trauma,
- vessels weakened by infection, e.g. septic
emboli from infective endocarditis (**mycotic
aneurysms**),
- coagulopathies.

Clinical features

Because blood irritates the meninges, the patient presents with sudden (seconds) very severe
headache with photophobia, nausea, vomiting
and signs of meningism (**neck stiffness** and
Kernig's sign, Chapter 9).

   With more severe haemorrhages, intracranial
pressure may rise and the level of consciousness deteriorate. Papilloedema and retinal haemorrhages
may be detectable on fundoscopy.

   Focal neurological signs may develop as a result
of:
- false localizing effect of raised intracranial pressure,
- coexistent intracerebral haemorrhage,
- spasm of vessels, as a result of the irritant effect
of blood, with concomitant ischaemia.

   Systemic features include bradycardia and hypertension, with rising intracranial pressure, and
fever possibly caused by hypothalamic damage.
Sometimes, subarachnoid haemorrhage may be
associated with pulmonary oedema and cardiac
arrhythmias.

Investigation

- CT cranial scan will reveal subarachnoid blood
in most cases (Fig. 11.7).
- Small bleeds may not be detectable on CT scan.
Lumbar puncture may be required to confirm the
diagnosis. There is no contraindication to this
once mass lesions have been excluded by imaging
and provided there is no bleeding diathesis.
- Lumbar puncture diagnostic of subarachnoid
haemorrhage typically shows frank blood that
fails to clear, i.e. all three bottles uniformly

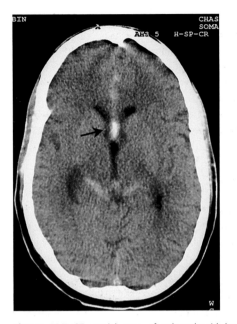

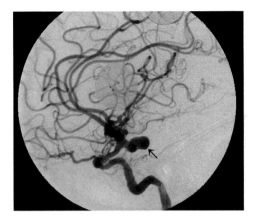

Figure 11.8 Carotid angiogram showing an aneurysm of the posterior communicating artery (arrowed).

Figure 11.7 CT cranial scan of subarachnoid haemorrhage. High-density areas, indicative of blood, are widespread but particularly evident in the interhemispheric fissure (arrowed) in this example of haemorrhage from an anterior communicating artery aneurysm.

bloodstained. The CSF supernatant is straw or yellow coloured (**xanthochromia**), within 3 hours of the haemorrhage, because of the presence of haemoglobin breakdown products.

• Pulmonary oedema and cardiac arrhythmias may be investigated by chest radiograph and electrocardiogram.

• Bleeding disorders should be excluded.

• Glycosuria is sometimes present.

Prognosis and management

Aneurysmal subarachnoid haemorrhage carries a very high mortality, 30–40% of patients dying in the first few days. There is a significant risk of rebleeding, particularly in the first 6 weeks, and the second bleed may be more severe than the first. Thus, management is directed towards immediate resuscitation of the patient and prevention of rebleeding.

Bed rest and analgesia are initially instituted. The calcium antagonist **nimodipine** has been shown to reduce early morbidity caused by ischaemia. Early complications of subarachnoid haemorrhage include **hydrocephalus** as a result of obstruction of CSF pathways by blood clot. This complication may also occur later (**communicating hydrocephalus**, Chapter 13). If the patient is alert or only mildly drowsy, investigation for the source of bleeding, by **cerebral angiography** (Fig. 11.8), should be performed at the earliest opportunity. Identification of an aneurysm may then permit early intervention. Operative techniques, such as **clipping** the aneurysmal neck or **wrapping** the aneurysm, have now been largely superseded by **endovascular** interventional neuroradiological approaches – occlusion of the aneurysm using detachable coils introduced by selective catheterisation.

The timing and advisability of angiography and intervention in patients with more severe subarachnoid haemorrhages and impairment of consciousness is a matter of specialist judgement, as these patients have a worse prognosis and tolerate treatment poorly.

Bleeding arteriovenous malformations have a lower mortality than aneurysms. Investigation is again by angiography and treatment may be by surgery, radiotherapy or interventional neuroradiology (Chapter 8). Arteriovenous malformations presenting without bleeding, e.g. with epilepsy, should not usually be treated surgically.

Spontaneous intracerebral haemorrhage

Haemorrhage into the substance of the brain may be caused by:
- hypertension, with microaneurysm formation (Charcot–Bouchard aneurysms),
- bleeding into tumours,
- trauma,
- blood disorders,
- blood vessel disorders – arteriovenous malformations, vasculitis, amyloid.

Intracerebral haemorrhage accounts for 10% of all strokes.

Patients present with focal neurological signs depending on the site of the bleed, seizures and features of raised intracranial pressure. The diagnosis is usually evident on CT scan.

Complications include hydrocephalus and **coning** (Chapter 13). Large haematomas hence have a poor prognosis (greater than 50% mortality), as do brainstem haemorrhages.

Treatment is initially medical with antihypertensive drugs, anti-epilepsy drugs for seizures, correction of coagulopathies and mannitol for raised intracranial pressure.

Surgical intervention includes:
- evacuation of haematoma – for cerebellar or cerebral lobar haemorrhages with progressive deterioration,
- ventricular drainage – for acute hydrocephalus (Chapter 13).

Key points

- Stroke is characterized by rapidly evolving clinical features due to loss of brain (or spinal cord) function; symptoms last more than 24 hours or lead to death
- Vascular mechanisms underlying stroke are either thromboembolic or haemorrhagic
- Stroke is the third most common cause of death in developed countries
- The clinical features of arterial brain infarcts depend on the vascular territory affected, the main distinction being between the anterior and posterior circulations
- CT cranial scan is useful in distinguishing between cerebral infarction and haemorrhage
- Up to 15% of patients with ischaemic stroke are eligible for thrombolysis
- Patients should be admitted to a specialist stroke unit
- Stroke prevention includes modifying risk factors, particularly smoking and hypertension
- Antiplatelet therapy should be started as soon as possible after a cerebral infarct
- Transient ischaemic attacks are most commonly due to embolism from neck vessels; treatment consists of modifying risk factors, antiplatelet therapy (or warfarin for cardiogenic embolism) and endarterectomy for severe symptomatic carotid stenoses
- Subarachnoid haemorrhage presents with meningism and can usually be diagnosed on CT scan

---

Transient ischaemic attack due to cardiogenic embolism

Case history: A 73-year-old man experienced an episode of weakness of his left arm and to a milder degree his left leg. His wife noticed that the left side of his face was drooping during the episode and his speech was slurred. All symptoms resolved within a few hours and neurological examination was normal by the time he was seen. However, his pulse was irregular and an electrocardiogram confirmed atrial fibrillation.

Comment: With a history compatible with an embolic event in right middle cerebral artery territory, in the presence of atrial fibrillation, this patient warrants lifelong anticoagulation provided brain imaging shows no evidence of haemorrhage and there is no other contraindication. It might be argued that his TIA was due to small vessel disease in situ in the brain, and was unrelated to his arrhythmia, which may not even have been present at the time of the cerebral event. However, the risk/benefit analysis is in favour of anticoagulation in this example. Having said this, due attention should also be paid to the management of this patient's other vascular risk factors.

Continued on p. 90

Subarachnoid haemorrhage

Case history: A 47-year-old woman developed a very severe headache of sudden onset. At her local casualty department, she was found to be fully conscious and apyrexial, but in pain, with moderate neck stiffness and photophobia. She had vomited once. There were no focal abnormal neurological signs. A CT cranial scan was thought to be normal. She was discharged home with a presumptive diagnosis of migraine (there was no antecedent history of headache) and analgesics. Two weeks later, she suffered an unexplained episode of loss of consciousness of uncertain duration – she lived alone and found herself on the bathroom floor when she regained consciousness, having vomited into the toilet bowl. Her general practitioner referred her to another hospital for a neurological opinion.

By the time she was seen in the neurology outpatient clinic, it was thought too late to examine her CSF for xanthochromia, despite her having been seen urgently. Repeat CT cranial scan was again normal. She was admitted urgently for cerebral angiography, which showed an aneurysm of the left posterior communicating artery. This was subsequently occluded successfully.

Comment: A normal CT scan does not exclude subarachnoid haemorrhage. With a high index of suspicion, as in this patient's case, lumbar puncture should have been carried out immediately, as soon as imaging had ruled out a mass lesion. The patient should not have been sent home from casualty and was fortunate to survive the presumed second bleed, which caused the episode of loss of consciousness.

Chapter 12

Parkinson's disease and other movement disorders

Parkinson's disease

Parkinson's disease is a degenerative condition primarily affecting extrapyramidal pathways where dopamine is the neurotransmitter, and characterized by the clinical triad of:
- akinesia – poverty of movement,
- rigidity,
- tremor – shaking back and forth, usually of the upper limbs.

Aetiology and pathogenesis

Although the ultimate cause of Parkinson's disease is unknown, other, generally rarer, **akinetic–rigid syndromes** have an identified aetiology (Table 12.1).

The recognition that MPTP, a synthetic heroin by-product, could produce acute Parkinsonism has provided some insight into the aetiology of Parkinson's disease itself (Fig. 12.1). The fact that an unusual exogenous toxin may lead to selective CNS damage and Parkinsonism has reinforced the view that idiopathic Parkinson's disease itself may be caused by exposure to a more widely prevalent environmental factor, as yet unidentified, perhaps

Lecture Notes: Neurology, 9th edition. By Lionel Ginsberg. Published 2010 by Blackwell Publishing.

acting by a similar mechanism to MPTP. Further support for environmental factors includes the following:
- The disease is increasingly common with age (mean age of onset about 60 years).
- Genetic causative factors have been identified but a positive family history is relatively unusual in idiopathic Parkinson's disease.
- There is a weak association between Parkinson's disease and various environmental factors, e.g. exposure to wood pulp and pesticides.

Epidemiology

Parkinson's disease is common, probably affecting about 1–2% of the population aged 60+ years, with no significant gender bias. It has a worldwide distribution, though it appears more common in Europe and North America.

Pathology

The dopaminergic neurones primarily affected in Parkinson's disease are those projecting from the substantia nigra of the midbrain to the striatum of the basal ganglia (caudate nucleus and putamen). Macroscopically, atrophy of the substantia nigra in advanced Parkinson's disease is recognizable by loss of the characteristic melanin pigmentation

Table 12.1 Causes of an akinetic–rigid syndrome.

Inherited
Wilson's disease – Chapter 18

Traumatic
'Punch-drunk syndrome' – chronic head injury in
   boxers – patients have parkinsonian features often
   in combination with cerebellar damage and
   cognitive deficits (dementia pugilistica)

Inflammatory
Postencephalitic Parkinsonism – following the
   epidemic of encephalitis lethargica after World War
   I, patients developed a chronic akinetic–rigid state,
   with certain characteristic features, particularly
   oculogyric crises (see text)

Neoplastic
Tumours of the basal ganglia presenting with
   contralateral hemiparkinsonism are extremely rare

Vascular
Multiple lacunar infarcts may occasionally result in
   pseudoparkinsonian features, but usually in
   association with pyramidal and cognitive dysfunction

Drugs
Neuroleptics
Antiemetics
Amiodarone

Toxins
MPTP
Manganese
Chronic carbon monoxide poisoning

Idiopathic
Parkinson's disease
(Other idiopathic syndromes are listed in Table 12.2)

of this region (Fig. 12.2). Microscopically, severe neuronal loss is demonstrable in the substantia nigra, remaining neurones often containing a distinctive intracellular inclusion, the **Lewy body** (Fig. 12.3). Symptoms of Parkinson's disease appear when about 60–80% of nigrostriate dopaminergic neurones have been lost.

Pathophysiologically, damage to dopaminergic pathways leads to an imbalance in the extrapyramidal system in favour of cholinergic and other neurotransmitter mechanisms (Fig. 12.4).

Clinical features

Akinesia

Patients with Parkinson's disease may complain that they have 'slowed down' physically (**bradykinesia**), experiencing particular difficulty with complex motor tasks, e.g. dressing, shaving, handwriting (which often becomes smaller – **micrographia**).

Lack of spontaneous movement may manifest itself by:
- poverty of facial expression, patients often being described as having an impassive or mask-like face,
- difficulty changing position, e.g. turning in bed,
- quiet and monotonous speech,
- abnormal gait and stance, partly as a consequence of akinesia and partly because of loss of normal postural control.

Gait

Patients typically adopt a flexed, or stooped, posture (Fig. 12.5), sometimes unkindly described as **simian** or apelike. They may be unable to maintain a normal stance in response to pressure from behind, the patient falling forward (**propulsion**), or from in front, falling backwards (**retropulsion**). Initiation of walking may be difficult ('**freezing**'), as may turning. Patients may use 'tricks' such as deliberately stepping over a walking stick to change direction or get through doorways. Steps are typically small and shuffling, the gait described as **festinant**, as if the patient is hurrying to keep up with his or her own centre of gravity. Normal arm swing on walking is lost. With severe postural instability in advanced Parkinson's disease, there is increasing risk of falls.

Rigidity

The increase in muscle tone in Parkinson's disease differs from spasticity (Chapter 5) by being relatively constant throughout the range of movement of the joint being tested – **lead pipe rigidity**.

Cogwheel rigidity may be regarded as a consequence of the tremor of Parkinson's disease being superimposed on background lead pipe

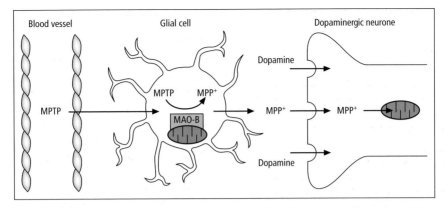

Figure 12.1 MPTP and the aetiology of Parkinson's disease. The toxin MPTP crosses the blood–brain barrier and is converted to its active metabolite MPP+ by the enzyme monoamine oxidase type B (MAO-B) in glial cells. MPP+, a free radical, is concentrated in dopaminergic neurones, entering via the dopamine reuptake mechanism, thereby selectively damaging these cells. MPP+ is a mitochondrial poison, inhibiting Complex I of the respiratory chain, and hence impairing cellular energy production.

rigidity. It is most frequently detected with repeated flexion and extension, or rotation, at the wrist. Rigidity in one arm can be accentuated by asking the patient simultaneously to lift and lower the opposite arm repeatedly.

Tremor

Tremor may be formally defined as an involuntary, repetitive, rhythmic sinusoidal movement usually affecting one or more limbs, but occasionally involving the head (**titubation**), face, jaw or trunk. In Parkinson's disease, the tremor:

- primarily affects the hands but may involve upper and lower limbs, and less frequently the jaw and lips, but not the head or neck,
- in the hands is often described as '**pill rolling**',
- has a characteristic frequency of 3–6 Hz,
- is present at rest and exacerbated by anxiety or stress,
- improves and may disappear on action.

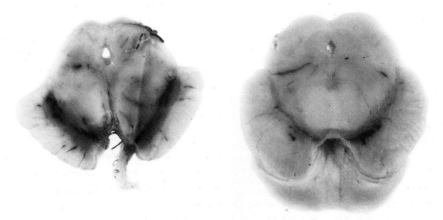

(a)

(b)

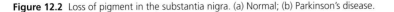

Figure 12.2 Loss of pigment in the substantia nigra. (a) Normal; (b) Parkinson's disease.

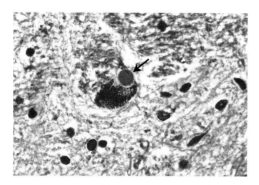

Figure 12.3 The Lewy body (arrowed).

Early in Parkinson's disease, tremor and other physical signs are typically markedly asymmetrical, even unilateral. A substantial minority of patients with Parkinson's disease display only akinesia and rigidity, without tremor. Other patients may have a postural tremor (see below) rather than a classical resting tremor.

Other motor symptoms and signs

• **Cranial nerves**. Examination of eye movements may reveal a mild impairment of upgaze. The eyelids may be tremulous (**blepharoclonus**). The 'glabellar tap sign' is elicited by repeated taps to the forehead. In unaffected individuals, re-flex blinking rapidly fatigues, whereas in Parkinson's disease there is a blink response each time the forehead is touched, without fatigue. However, the sign is far from specific for Parkinson's disease.

• Difficulty swallowing, including the patient's own saliva, may result in a tendency to drool (**sialorrhoea**).

• **Limbs**. Muscle power, tendon reflexes and sensation are normal; plantar responses are downgoing. Pain or aching in muscles is common – many patients present with, or develop, a 'frozen shoulder'.

Non-motor symptoms

• **Depression** is common and may arise independently of the degree of motor dysfunction.

• **Hallucinations**. Vivid, formed visual hallucinations may occur, particularly at night, and need not necessarily indicate cognitive impairment or psychosis.

• **Psychosis**. Worsening hallucinations and delusions may escalate to full-blown psychosis, particularly in patients who also have cognitive impairment.

• **Dementia**. Cognitive impairment (Chapters 3 and 18) is a common accompaniment of advanced Parkinson's disease.

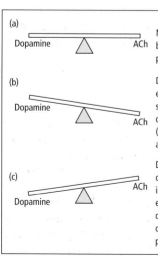

(a)
Dopamine — ACh
Normal-dopaminergic pathways balanced by those utilizing other neurotransmitters, predominantly acetylcholine (ACh).

(b)
Dopamine — ACh
Dopaminergic deficiency or cholinergic excess, resulting in an akinetic–rigid syndrome, e.g. idiopathic Parkinson's disease or drug-induced Parkinsonism (NB phenothiazines and related drugs are dopamine antagonists).

(c)
Dopamine — ACh
Dopaminergic excess or cholinergic deficiency, resulting in excessive involuntary movements – dyskinesia, e.g. due to overtreatment of Parkinson's disease with dopaminergic drugs, or to degenerative disease of non-dopaminergic pathways, as in Huntington's disease.

Figure 12.4 The concept of neuro-chemical balance in the extrapyramidal system.

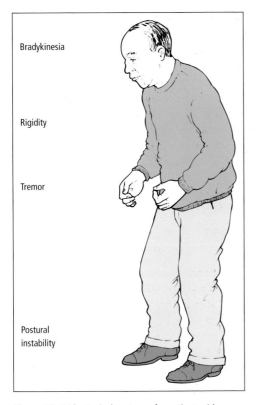

Bradykinesia

Rigidity

Tremor

Postural
instability

Figure 12.5 The typical posture of a patient with Parkinson's disease.

• **Sleep disorder**. Insomnia is common in Parkinson's disease and may relate to immobility, mood disturbance, hallucinations and various sleep-related behavioural and movement disorders.
• **Autonomic symptoms**. The skin may have a greasy **seborrhoeic** texture. Constipation is common, as are bladder disturbance and erectile dysfunction. Other autonomic features, e.g. postural hypotension, are relatively milder than in multiple system atrophy (Table 12.2), but still occur commonly in advanced Parkinson's disease.
• **Anosmia** is a feature of Parkinson's disease which may antedate the onset of motor dysfunction by many years.

Course and prognosis

Parkinson's disease is progressive. It may be divided into three stages – early, when symp-

Table 12.2 Idiopathic akinetic–rigid syndromes other than Parkinson's disease.

Multiple system atrophy (MSA)
Extrapyramidal features in combination with one or more of the following:
    Autonomic failure (Shy–Drager syndrome)
    Cerebellar dysfunction
    Pyramidal features
When Parkinsonism predominates, the syndrome is termed MSA-P as opposed to MSA-C when cerebellar features predominate and MSA-A when autonomic failure is pronounced

Progressive supranuclear palsy (PSP, Steele–Richardson–Olszewski syndrome)
Failure of voluntary gaze – first downgaze, then upgaze, then horizontal gaze – associated with extrapyramidal dysfunction (with early postural instability) and dementia

Syndromes combining parkinsonian features with cerebral cortical dysfunction (Chapter 18)
Corticobasal degeneration (CBD) – extremely rare
Dementia with Lewy bodies (DLB)

tom control is good; mid, when motor fluctuations and dyskinesias (see below) develop; and late, when treatment-resistant features, such as dementia and falls, occur. Untreated patients used to reach a severely disabling degree of immobility, with threat to life from the risk of bronchopneumonia, septicaemia or pulmonary embolus, after 7–10 years of disease on average. Current treatments are largely symptomatic but probably have also improved average life expectancy.

Diagnosis

• The diagnosis of Parkinson's disease is based on the presence of the triad of clinical features. Asymmetry of signs at onset is important.
• Brain imaging by standard CT or MR techniques is unhelpful.
• PET scanning (Chapter 8) is at present purely a research tool and is not routinely available for the vast majority of patients. Dopamine transporter (DaT) SPECT scans can reveal a nigrostriate

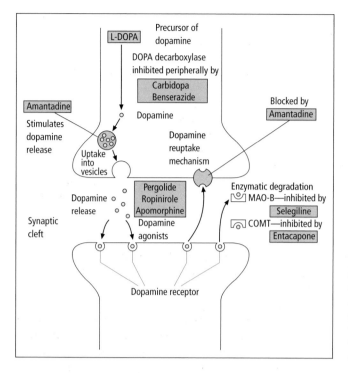

Figure 12.6 Actions of drugs which improve dopaminergic transmission in Parkinson's disease. Amantadine, a weak antiparkinsonian drug, appears to act by several mechanisms. In addition to those illustrated which relate directly to dopaminergic transmission, there are also indirect effects via pathways utilizing other neurotransmitters, e.g. glutamate.

dopaminergic lesion, but the changes are not specific to idiopathic Parkinson's disease and may be found in other akinetic–rigid syndromes.

• Where the diagnosis is in doubt, a patient's response to drug treatment (see below) may be informative.

Most of the causes of an akinetic–rigid syndrome (Table 12.1) will be readily distinguishable from idiopathic Parkinson's disease by the clinical features and relevant investigations (drug-induced Parkinsonism is an important differential diagnosis). However, there are other idiopathic akinetic–rigid syndromes (Table 12.2) that may be more difficult to diagnose, a lack of response to antiparkinsonian treatment being an important discriminant. Having said this, some patients with multiple system atrophy will respond to such treatment, at least initially. Parkinson's disease must also be distinguished from other causes of tremor (see below), from cerebrovascular disease and from normal-pressure hydrocephalus (Chapters 13 and 18).

Treatment

Drug therapy

This is largely symptomatic and aimed at restoring the neurochemical balance (Fig. 12.4) either by anticholinergic agents or, more importantly, with drugs that enhance the dopaminergic pathway (Fig. 12.6). Treatment is best delayed until symptoms warrant it.

L-DOPA

This is the mainstay of drug treatment for Parkinson's disease severe enough to cause significant functional disability. It is the natural substrate for the synthesis of dopamine (Fig. 12.7). Unlike dopamine itself, L-DOPA is able to cross the blood–brain barrier and can, therefore, reach its site of action following oral administration.

However, most of an oral dose of L-DOPA is metabolized to dopamine by peripheral DOPA decarboxylase before reaching the brain. It is therefore generally given in combination with a peripheral

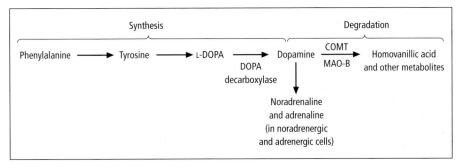

Figure 12.7 Pathways of dopamine metabolism. In addition to enzymatic degradation by monoamine oxidase type B (MAO-B) and catechol-*O*-methyltransferase (COMT), dopamine is also removed from synaptic clefts by a selective reuptake mechanism into neurones.

DOPA decarboxylase inhibitor (**benserazide** or **carbidopa**). This has the additional benefit of reducing peripheral side effects of L-DOPA (nausea, vomiting), which may also be limited by gradual escalation of the dose of L-DOPA in accordance with symptoms.

Co-careldopa (L-DOPA plus carbidopa) and **co-beneldopa** (L-DOPA plus benserazide) may have central side effects (postural hypotension, confusion, hallucinations, delusions), but most patients with idiopathic Parkinson's disease benefit from their use at least early in the disease.

Complications of long-term L-DOPA therapy in Parkinson's disease
Unfortunately, after 2–5 years, the efficacy of L-DOPA becomes limited by the complications of **motor fluctuations** and **dyskinesias**.

Motor fluctuations are:
• 'wearing-off', where individual doses produce only short-lived effects,
• 'on–off', where the patient may switch from symptomatic benefit from medication ('on') to an akinetic–rigid state ('off'), often without any predictable relationship to the timing of drug doses.

Dyskinesias are involuntary movements occurring in association with drug treatment, e.g. twisting, turning movements when dopamine levels are high ('**peak-dose dyskinesias**'), or painful sustained muscle contractions, typically of the feet, when dopamine levels are low

('**wearing-off dystonias**'). Some patients are prepared to tolerate moderate dyskinesias if they can remain mobile.

A small proportion of patients with Parkinson's disease seem to crave L-DOPA at doses well above that required for motor function, with resulting bizarre, repetitive, compulsive behavioural disturbances (dopamine dysregulation syndrome).

Motor fluctuations and dyskinesias can be partially alleviated in some patients by:
• frequent small doses of L-DOPA-containing drugs,
• controlled release preparations,
• the combined use of L-DOPA-containing preparations with **selegiline**, a monoamine oxidase type B (MAO-B) inhibitor (which blocks dopamine metabolism), **entacapone**, a catechol-*O*-methyltransferase (COMT) inhibitor (which blocks L-DOPA metabolism), or direct **dopamine receptor agonists** (see below). **Tolcapone** is another COMT inhibitor, but its use has been restricted by the very rare occurrence of severe liver failure, which can prove fatal.
• attempts to mimic physiological dopamine levels by continuous administration of L-DOPA or dopamine agonists, as opposed to the intermittent nature of oral therapy. Such approaches include transdermal administration of **rotigotine**, a dopamine agonist, subcutaneous infusion of **apomorphine**, another agonist, and duodenal infusion of L-DOPA.
• surgery (see below).

Other side effects of L-DOPA are best treated by drugs with the least central dopamine antagonist action, e.g. **domperidone** for nausea, and **'atypical neuroleptics'** such as **risperidone, olanzapine, quetiapine** and **clozapine**, or **cholinesterase inhibitors** (Chapter 18), such as **donepezil** and **rivastigmine**, for hallucinations in patients with cognitive impairment.

Other drugs

Selegiline may have a further role as sole treatment in early Parkinson's disease. On theoretical grounds, it might be predicted to slow the progression of the disease by inhibiting MAO-B and thereby potentially blocking the conversion of a putative environmental pro-toxin analogous to MPTP to its activated, free radical, form. This **neuroprotective** mechanism remains controversial. However, many neurologists treat patients with early Parkinson's disease, and insufficient functional disability to warrant L-DOPA, with selegiline alone. It may delay the requirement for L-DOPA by up to 12 months, though this could be through a mild dopaminergic action of its own. **Rasagiline** is a newer MAO-B inhibitor.

Dopamine agonists include **bromocriptine, cabergoline, pergolide, ropinirole,· pramipexole, rotigotine** and **apomorphine**. These drugs also have an important role in early Parkinson's disease, potentially delaying the need for L-DOPA, and hence delaying and possibly reducing the frequency of its long-term motor complications. Many neurologists now advise that agonists alone are used initially to treat Parkinson's disease, particularly in younger patients who are more at risk of developing DOPA-induced dyskinesias and fluctuations earlier and to a more severe degree. The first three drugs listed are derived from ergot, and are associated with pulmonary and retroperitoneal fibrosis. Up to one-third of patients on pergolide develop fibrotic cardiac valvulopathy. For this reason, non-ergoline dopamine agonists are preferred nowadays. However, ropinirole and pramipexole also have adverse effects, which include excessive drowsiness, even sudden onset of sleep without warning, and bizarre behavioural disturbances such as pathological gambling.

Amantadine, despite the theoretical appeal of its probable mechanisms of action (Fig. 12.6), is only mildly beneficial in early Parkinson's disease. Later, it can reduce L-DOPA-induced dyskinesias, albeit only for a limited period, typically 6–9 months.

Anticholinergic drugs, such as trihexyphenidyl, orphenadrine and benztropine, also produce only minor benefits, though they are said to help tremor, against which L-DOPA preparations are less useful. However, the anticholinergic drugs have serious side effects peripherally, e.g. urinary retention, dry mouth, blurred vision, and centrally, particularly confusion and hallucinations in the elderly.

Therapeutic trials

The response to treatment can be useful in the diagnosis of Parkinson's disease, as most patients with idiopathic Parkinson's disease will improve with pharmacological enhancing of dopaminergic transmission. This can be assessed on an outpatient basis by the patient completing a diary of periods 'on' and 'off' after the introduction of L-DOPA-containing preparations. Diaries may also help with manipulating the subsequent timing and dosage of these drugs. An alternative diagnostic approach is to observe a patient's motor function (e.g., timed walking) before and for several hours after a single large dose of an L-DOPA-containing preparation, or after administration of a dopamine receptor agonist (incremental doses of subcutaneous apomorphine may be used for this purpose in specialist centres).

Surgical treatment

Stereotactic thalamotomy (a surgical lesion to the thalamus) is infrequently used with improved drug therapy, though it has a role in patients with severe tremor unresponsive to medication.

A more modern approach is to interrupt the output of the subthalamic nucleus or the globus pallidus (pars interna), either by a lesion or using an implanted deep brain stimulation device. These nuclei are overactive as a result of the neurochemical imbalance, and such functional neurosurgical techniques have a role in the treatment of dyskinesias and motor fluctuations.

Cell transplantation using fetal substantia nigra is still an experimental technique. Its role in idiopathic Parkinson's disease is not established, though patients with MPTP-induced Parkinsonism have shown more marked improvement.

Other movement disorders – dyskinesias

These represent the opposite pole of the spectrum of movement disorders to akinetic–rigid syndromes. Excessive involuntary movements may be encountered as a consequence of drug treatment of Parkinson's disease, as described previously, but there are many other causes.

Chorea

Choreiform movements are irregular, random and variable but have a flowing or 'dancing' quality, which may appear semipurposeful. Any part of the body may be affected, normal movement being interrupted by chorea. Causes of acquired chorea other than chronic L-DOPA therapy in Parkinson's disease include:
- postinfectious (**Sydenham's chorea** in association with rheumatic fever, now rarely seen),
- polycythaemia rubra vera,
- systemic lupus erythematosus,
- thyrotoxicosis,
- pregnancy and the oral contraceptive,
- phenytoin, alcohol, neuroleptics.

Hereditary chorea is seen in **Huntington's disease** (Chapter 18) in association with dementia, but may also occur in other rare inherited disorders.

Chorea may respond to the monoamine-depleting drug **tetrabenazine**, but this may produce severe depression. Alternatives include neuroleptics, e.g. sulpiride or haloperidol.

In **hemiballismus**, the movements are more violent and jerky, and are restricted to one side of the body, occurring as a result of damage to the contralateral **subthalamic nucleus**.

Athetosis

These movements are slower and more 'writhing' in quality than chorea. Athetosis represents the transition from one dystonic posture to another (see below). Typically, it is associated with congenital brain damage (cerebral palsy, Chapter 18), particularly that which used to occur with neonatal hyperbilirubinaemia (**kernicterus**).

Tremor

Causes of tremor other than Parkinson's disease are listed in Table 12.3.

Essential tremor is a common condition typically characterized by:
- positive family history,
- postural tremor of both hands, hence difficulty holding cups, writing, etc., but other body parts including the head (titubation) may be affected; tremor absent at rest,
- no extrapyramidal or cerebellar clinical features,
- tremor may be relieved by alcohol,
- may respond to treatment with propranolol or primidone.

Table 12.3 Causes of tremor.

Rest tremor
Parkinson's disease
Other akinetic–rigid syndromes
Postural tremor (maximal with maintained posture)
Essential tremor
Physiological tremor; may be exaggerated by:
Anxiety
Thyrotoxicosis
Alcohol
Drugs, e.g. bronchodilators
Kinetic tremor (i.e., during movement, often worse as a target is approached – intention tremor)
Cerebellar diseases:
Multiple sclerosis
Hereditary ataxias
Tumour, infarct or haemorrhage of the cerebellum
Postural and kinetic tremors may be associated with dystonia, and with some peripheral neuropathies

Primary orthostatic tremor presents with unsteadiness or tremor in the legs, brought on by prolonged standing. Clonazepam can be helpful.

Dystonia

Involuntary sustained muscle contractions resulting in abnormal postures may be subclassified as:
- Focal, e.g.
  - **blepharospasm** – involuntary eye closure,
  - **oculogyric crisis** – eyes rolled upwards, as seen in postencephalitic Parkinsonism,
  - **spasmodic torticollis** – 'wry neck', painful contraction of sternomastoid, which may hypertrophy (and other neck muscles), resulting in head being turned involuntarily to one side, also sometimes forwards (**antecollis**) or backwards (**retrocollis**),
  - **laryngospasm** – with stridor,
  - **trismus** – jaw spasm,
  - **writer's cramp** – painful, abnormal posture of the hand stopping the patient writing, characteristically task-specific;
- Generalized: as in the inherited condition of **primary torsion dystonia** (formerly known as dystonia musculorum deformans) but also seen in drug reactions and as a symptom of many causes of cerebral damage, e.g. anoxia.

Drug treatment is generally unsatisfactory, though generalized dystonias may respond to increasing doses of anticholinergic agents, e.g. trihexyphenidyl. One rare form of inherited dystonia, typically presenting in the lower limbs in childhood, is strikingly responsive to modest doses of L-DOPA. Focal dystonias may be successfully treated by injection of affected muscles with **botulinum toxin**, in specialist centres. Rare **paroxysmal dystonias** may respond to anti-epilepsy drugs.

Myoclonus

These are rapid, abrupt, jerky, 'shock-like' movements of part or the whole of the body, which may occur in the context of abnormal electrical discharges of the cerebral cortex, hence an association with epilepsy (Chapter 10). However, myoclonic jerks can also arise from elsewhere in the CNS, including the spinal cord, and may feature in degenerative and metabolic brain disorders. Sodium valproate and clonazepam are first-line drugs for myoclonic epilepsies.

Tics

These are rapid, compulsive, repetitive, stereotyped movements, therefore also known as '**habit spasms**'. The movement can be voluntarily resisted for a limited period, but often is more violent immediately after resistance has been abandoned.

In **Gilles de la Tourette syndrome**, complex tics are associated with involuntary utterances, which are often repetitive (**echolalia**) and obscene (**coprolalia**). Drug treatment is difficult but patients may respond to neuroleptics.

Drug-induced movement disorders

Many drugs may induce tremor (Table 12.3).

Neuroleptic drugs, not surprisingly through their dopamine receptor antagonist action, are associated with many motor side effects, including:
- acute dystonic reactions,
- **akathisia** – restlessness, the patient typically seeming 'jittery' and unable to sit down,
- drug-induced Parkinsonism,
- **tardive dyskinesia** – in which patients develop involuntary movements, especially of the face and mouth, which may persist after the neuroleptic drug has been discontinued.

The most severe movement disorder seen with neuroleptics is the potentially life-threatening **neuroleptic malignant syndrome**, where patients have generalized muscular rigidity and fever in association with tremor, incontinence, altered consciousness and cardiovascular changes. The rigidity is sufficient to produce muscle damage with elevation of serum creatine kinase activity and sometimes myoglobinuria. Treatment, in addition to resuscitative measures and withdrawal of the offending drug, includes attempting to redress the neurochemical balance with a dopamine receptor agonist – bromocriptine – and use of a muscle relaxant – dantrolene.

Miscellaneous movement disorders

- **Restless legs syndrome**, also known as Ekbom's syndrome, is a common disorder in which patients have a distressing, irresistible desire to move the legs (akathisia), associated with an uncomfortable deep-seated sensation in the legs, worse in the evening or at night. The symptoms are brought on by rest and relieved by movement. Early-onset disease is often familial. The more usual presentation is an older female patient, with no family history, who may have signs of an underlying peripheral neuropathy (Chapter 17). Other associations include lumbar root disease (Chapter 15), iron deficiency and renal failure. If the problem is severe enough to warrant drug therapy, first-line treatment is with dopaminergic agents, either dopamine receptor agonists or L-DOPA. Other drugs include opiates, clonazepam, gabapentin and iron replacement therapy where appropriate. The syndrome of 'painful legs and moving toes' is much rarer than restless legs syndrome and harder to treat. These patients have more severe pain in the legs associated with involuntary continuous writhing movements of the toes. Again, there may be underlying disease of the lumbar roots or peripheral nerves.

- **Stiff person syndrome** is a very rare condition of slowly progressive rigidity of the trunk and proximal limbs, with superimposed painful muscle spasms. There is an association with diabetes and epilepsy. The diagnosis may be supported by characteristic EMG findings, the presence of specific auto-antibodies in some cases and of oligoclonal bands in the CSF (Chapter 16). In keeping with its presumed autoimmune basis, some patients with stiff person syndrome respond to immunomodulatory measures such as steroids, intravenous immunoglobulin or plasma exchange. Others benefit from symptomatic treatment, e.g. with benzodiazepines. There are other, more rapidly progressive, forms of spinal rigidity, some of which may be paraneoplastic.

- **Hemifacial spasm** is described in Chapter 4.

- **Psychogenic movement disorders** should be diagnosed with caution. A psychogenic basis may be suspected if a patient's movements are unusually variable, disappear with distraction and are associated with other clinical features suggesting a 'non-organic' cause (Chapter 19).

Key points

- Parkinson's disease:
  - is characterized by the clinical triad of akinesia, rigidity and tremor; patients may develop postural instability
  - is due to degeneration of nigrostriate dopaminergic neurones, with characteristic intracellular inclusions (Lewy bodies)
- The mainstay of drug treatment is L-DOPA, though late motor complications may develop with this therapy
- Dyskinesias (e.g., chorea) represent the opposite end of the movement disorder spectrum to akinetic–rigid syndromes

---

Parkinson's disease

Case history: A 61-year-old man reported a 6-month history of tremor affecting his left hand, with no other symptoms. Examination showed an impassive facial expression, a 'pill-rolling' tremor of the left hand, present at rest and disappearing on action, and cogwheel rigidity at the left wrist. He had a mildly flexed posture with reduced arm swing on the left when walking.

Comment: The presence of all three components of the classical clinical triad – rest tremor, rigidity and bradykinesia (impassive face, impaired arm swing) – indicates a diagnosis of early idiopathic Parkinson's disease. The asymmetry of this patient's presentation provides further support for this diagnosis. Clinical features, in addition to symmetrical onset, which point towards akinetic–rigid syndromes other than idiopathic Parkinson's disease, include the presence of significant postural hypotension. Though patients with idiopathic Parkinson's disease may have a mild postural drop in blood pressure, it is usually much more evident in multiple system atrophy (Shy–Drager syndrome). Eye movements should also be examined carefully. Though patients with idiopathic Parkinson's disease may have mild impairment of upgaze, a more marked vertical gaze palsy, including downgaze impairment, suggests a diagnosis of progressive supranuclear palsy (Steele–Richardson–Olszewski syndrome).

Chapter 13

Neurosurgical topics: head injury and brain tumour

General principles

Raised intracranial pressure

The clinical features of a chronic increase in intracranial pressure (headache, vomiting, papilloedema) have been described in detail in Chapter 9. When pressure rises acutely, additional physical signs supervene, dependent on the location of any expanding mass (Fig. 13.1). Acute increases in pressure may result, for example, from an intracranial haematoma caused by trauma, or when there is acute-on-chronic deterioration as a result of a tumour reaching a critical size and 'decompensating' (Fig. 13.2). Ultimately, with herniation of brain tissue through the tentorium or foramen magnum, there is potentially lethal compression of the brainstem, at either midbrain or medullary level ('**coning**').

Hydrocephalus

Rising intracranial pressure, caused by an expanding mass within the enclosed confines of the cranium, may be exacerbated if the normal pathway for CSF flow is obstructed by the mass (Fig. 13.3). This is because the site of CSF production (the choroid plexus in the cerebral ventricles) becomes disconnected from its site of absorption (the arachnoid villi, contiguous with the subarachnoid space), with resultant ventricular dilatation (Fig. 13.4).

Hydrocephalus, or an increase in CSF volume, is classified as:
- **obstructive** – if CSF flow is blocked within the ventricles. This may arise from congenital abnormalities (e.g., cerebral aqueduct stenosis, Arnold–Chiari malformation – Chapter 18) as well as mass lesions (tumour or haematoma). Acute obstructive hydrocephalus requires urgent surgical management, excess CSF being removed by a **ventricular drain**, or, as permanent management, being redirected to another body cavity (e.g., **ventriculoperitoneal shunting**);
- **communicating** – if CSF flow is blocked 'beyond' the ventricular system, e.g., as a result of damage to the meninges and hence also the arachnoid villi themselves:
  - meningitis (Chapter 14),
  - subarachnoid haemorrhage (Chapter 11) (both these may also cause obstructive hydrocephalus),

or if CSF viscosity is increased as a result of high protein concentration.

Other forms of hydrocephalus with particular clinical features and management aspects include:
- infantile hydrocephalus (Chapter 18),
- 'normal-pressure' hydrocephalus (Chapter 18).

Lecture Notes: Neurology, 9th edition. By Lionel Ginsberg. Published 2010 by Blackwell Publishing.

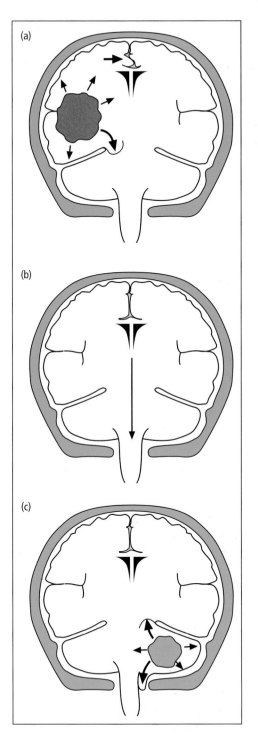

Cerebral oedema

A further mechanism that may contribute to the increase in intracranial pressure produced by an expanding mass lesion is the tendency for excess brain water to accumulate around such a lesion, thereby adding to the '**space-occupying**' effect. Cerebral oedema may be extracellular (**vasogenic**) or intracellular (**cytotoxic**) – Chapter 11.

Head injury

Aetiology and pathology

The causes of head trauma are listed in Table 13.1. By far the most important cause of serious head injury is road accidents (60% of deaths caused by road accidents are a result of head injuries); alcohol is frequently a contributory factor.

Figure 13.1 Consequences of acute raised intracranial pressure dependent on site of lesion. (a) Cerebral hemisphere mass – initially causing lateral tentorial herniation (lower large arrow) as well as shift of midline structures (upper large arrow). In lateral tentorial herniation, the temporal lobe herniates through the tentorial hiatus. Compression of the reticular formation results in a deteriorating level of consciousness. A third nerve palsy due to compression of both the nerve and the oculomotor nucleus in the midbrain manifests as an ipsilateral fixed (i.e., unresponsive to light) dilated pupil. There may also be long tract signs, e.g. upgoing plantar responses. (b) Central tentorial herniation – diffuse cerebral swelling, or unchecked lateral herniation, may result in vertical displacement of structures through the tentorial hiatus (arrowed). Conscious level deteriorates; pupils are initially small, ultimately fixed and moderately dilated. Other features include impaired upgaze due to pressure on the superior midbrain and associated structures, and diabetes insipidus due to downward traction on the pituitary stalk and hypothalamus. (c) Tonsillar herniation – due to a subtentorial mass or unchecked tentorial herniation. The cerebellar tonsils herniate through the foramen magnum (lower large arrow). A posterior fossa mass may also cause upward herniation through the tentorial hiatus (upper large arrow). Tonsillar herniation produces neck rigidity and sometimes a head tilt (particularly in children). Conscious level deteriorates, ultimately with respiratory arrest. Vital signs may be affected – hypertension and bradycardia.

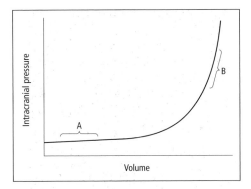

Figure 13.2 Decompensation of an expanding intracranial mass lesion. Initial expansion does not affect intracranial pressure significantly due to compensatory mechanisms (region A). Eventually, however, small increments in volume produce marked changes in pressure (region B).

Brain damage as a result of head injury arises from two related mechanisms:

- **Damage at impact**
  - **contusion** and **laceration** of cerebral cortex, usually frontal and temporal lobes, at site of impact, or opposite side ('**contre-coup**' injury),
  - diffuse white matter lesions as a result of **axonal shearing** and disruption consequent on deceleration (**diffuse axonal injury**);
- **Secondary complications**
  - haematoma (extradural, subdural, intracerebral),
  - cerebral oedema,

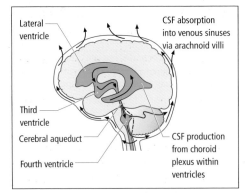

Figure 13.3 Pathway of normal CSF production, flow and absorption. Secreted by the choroid plexus, CSF normally flows from the ventricular system to the subarachnoid space via foramina in the fourth ventricle. It is absorbed into the venous system by the arachnoid villi.

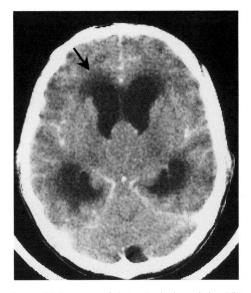

Figure 13.4 CT scan of obstructive hydrocephalus. Dilated lateral ventricles with periventricular lucency (low density – arrowed) indicating white matter oedema. A mass at the level of the third ventricle is blocking outflow from the lateral ventricles.

- cerebral ischaemia,
- coning,
- infection.

Unlike impact damage, these secondary complications may be readily treatable.

Clinical features

Head injury, particularly in road traffic accidents, frequently occurs in the context of multiple other injuries, which may take precedence in the immediate resuscitative management of the patient:

- **A**irway – with special care of the cervical spine, in case of coexistent fracture and/or dislocation,
- **B**reathing,

Table 13.1 Causes of head trauma.

Road traffic accidents
Falls
Assault – blunt injuries
Industrial injuries
Domestic accidents
Sporting accidents
Missile injuries – bullets and bomb fragments

- **C**irculation,
- major chest injury (haemothorax, pneumothorax),
- major abdominal bleeding.

Only after these aspects have been checked and corrected can the patient be assessed for head, spinal and finally limb injuries.

The history in head-injured patients is frequently obtained from witnesses. Important considerations include:
- Circumstances of injury – the patient may have suffered the injury as a consequence of prior loss of consciousness, e.g. as a result of a convulsion.
- Duration of period of loss of consciousness and of post-traumatic amnesia. The presence of a **'lucid interval'** between an initial period of loss of consciousness at the time of impact and the patient's level of consciousness subsequently deteriorating again strongly suggests the development of a potentially treatable secondary complication, i.e. intracranial haematoma.
- Persistence of headache and vomiting – may signify an intracranial haematoma.

The main components of the neurological examination of a head-injured patient are:
- external evidence of trauma
  - lacerations and bruising;
- signs of basal skull fracture
  - bilateral periorbital haematoma, haematoma over mastoid (**Battle's sign**),
  - subconjunctival haematoma – blood under conjunctiva with no posterior margin, indicating blood tracking forwards from orbit,
  - CSF discharge from nose or ear (clear, colourless fluid, positive for glucose),
  - bleeding from ear;
- level of consciousness (Glasgow Coma Scale),
- remainder of neurological examination, particularly pupillary responses, looking for signs of incipient tentorial herniation.

Investigations

- Skull radiograph, for fractures, if the patient has transient or persistent impairment of consciousness following the injury, external physical signs suggesting basal, vault or facial fracture, or focal

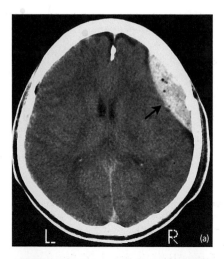

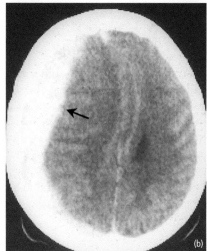

Figure 13.5 CT scans of acute traumatic intracranial haematomas (arrowed). (a) Extradural. Note the small, circular, very low density abnormalities within the haematoma. These are air bubbles, indicating that the haematoma is associated with a compound fracture. (b) Subdural. Trauma may also be associated with subarachnoid and intracerebral bleeding.

neurological signs. A skull fracture in the temporoparietal region in an unconscious patient suggests a possible extradural haematoma, caused by tearing of the middle meningeal artery.
- CT cranial scan (Fig. 13.5), required urgently if level of consciousness is deteriorating or if the patient has a skull fracture in combination with confusion, seizures or focal neurological signs.

Management

In general, there should be a low threshold for admission to hospital for observation after head injury. Admission is essential in the presence of:

- depressed conscious level,
- skull fracture,
- focal neurological signs.

Minor head injuries are managed solely by neurological observation, and cleansing and suturing of scalp lacerations. For more severe head injuries, specialist neurosurgical management is required after immediate resuscitative measures.

Specific aspects of treatment of severe head injury may be summarized into two categories, as follows.

Surgical

- Intracranial – urgent neurosurgical evacuation of space-occupying haematoma.
- Extracranial – inspection for compound depressed skull fracture underlying scalp laceration. If present, this requires urgent (within 24 hours) neurosurgical treatment by wound debridement and elevation of bone fragments to prevent subsequent infection of meninges and brain.

Medical

- Intravenous **mannitol** bolus (20%; 100 mL) for raised intracranial pressure. This may be required as an emergency measure before evacuation of intracranial haematoma in a patient with deteriorating level of consciousness. Patients with cerebral swelling but no identifiable haematoma may require repeated boluses of mannitol and possibly elective artificial **hyperventilation** in conjunction with continuous intracranial pressure monitoring.
- **Prophylactic antibiotics** for basal skull fracture.
- **Anti-epileptic drugs** for seizures.
- Sedative and narcotic drugs are contraindicated, as they may further depress conscious level.

Complications and consequences of head injury

- **Sequelae of severe head injury.** Even after severe trauma, most survivors regain independence. Some, however, are disabled both physically (dysphasia, hemiparesis, cranial nerve palsies) and mentally (cognitive impairment, altered personality). A small number remain in a permanent **vegetative state**. Head injury remains a significant cause of death (9 per 100,000 of the population per year), particularly in the young.
- **CSF leakage.** This may be present from the time of injury, but if the communication between the subarachnoid space and the middle ear or paranasal sinuses resulting from a basal fracture is small, and plugged by brain tissue, overt leakage may be absent and the patient may present late with meningitis. In addition to treatment of the infection, this complication requires surgical repair of the dural tear. Surgical exploration is also warranted if overt CSF leakage persists.
- **Post-traumatic epilepsy.** Particularly if the patient experiences early seizures (within the first week after injury), prolonged post-traumatic amnesia (more than 24 hours), a depressed skull fracture or an intracranial haematoma.
- **Post-concussion syndrome.** Headache, vertigo, depression and impaired concentration may persist even after minor head injury. Vertigo may be a consequence of vestibular trauma ('**labyrinthine concussion**').
- **Chronic subdural haematoma.** This late complication of head trauma (the injury may be minor) is described in more detail in the differential diagnosis of dementia (Chapter 18).

Brain tumour

Pathology

Intracranial neoplasms may be classified as:

- Benign – generally extra-axial, i.e. arising from meninges, cranial nerves or other structures and exerting extrinsic compression on brain substance. Though histologically 'benign', these tumours may be life-threatening because of space occupation within the confines of the cranial cavity.

- Malignant – generally intra-axial, i.e. arising within brain parenchyma:
  - primary – commonly of glial cell origin (**gliomas**) (these tumours are classified as malignant because of their local invasive properties, metastasis to extracranial sites is very rare, various histological subtypes and grades of differentiation are recognized),
  - secondary – metastases from malignant tumours elsewhere in the body.

Primary malignant brain tumours account for more than half of adult intracranial neoplasms; brain metastases make up 15–20% of intracranial tumours.

Clinical features and investigation

Malignant brain tumours have three main modes of presentation, which may occur in combination:

- epilepsy,
- raised intracranial pressure – usually a chronic course with headache, vomiting and papilloedema, but ultimately acute deterioration may occur with coning,
- focal neurological deficit, e.g. dysphasia, hemiparesis, cerebellar ataxia, visual field defects, cognitive impairment, personality change.

The investigation of suspected brain tumour has been revolutionized by the advent of sophisticated non-invasive imaging with CT or MR scans (Fig. 13.6). Other investigations include screening for primary neoplasm in a patient presenting with brain metastases, particularly by chest radiography.

Specific benign tumour syndromes

Meningioma

Benign meningeal tumours may present in similar ways to malignant brain neoplasms if arising from the meninges of the skull vault ('convexity' meningioma, Fig. 13.7), i.e. with epilepsy, raised intracranial pressure, dysphasia, hemiparesis and dementia. However, meningiomas growing in cer-

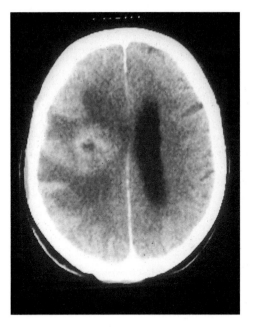

Figure 13.6 Cerebral glioma.

tain intracranial regions have more specific modes of presentation:

- Olfactory groove – unilateral then bilateral anosmia, papilloedema, frontal lobe dysfunction.
- Parasagittal region – spastic paraparesis mimicking a spinal cord lesion. UMN signs develop in

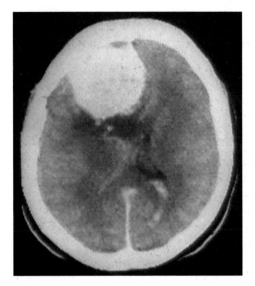

Figure 13.7 Intracranial meningioma.

both legs because the tumour is located between the cerebral hemispheres, compressing both motor homunculi in the region where the leg is represented.

- Cavernous sinus – with unilateral ophthalmoplegia (III, IV and VI palsies) and trigeminal sensory loss (ophthalmic and sometimes maxillary).
- Optic nerve – some meningiomas of the sphenoid wing may compress the optic nerve with unilateral visual failure and optic atrophy. Subsequent expansion of the tumour and hence raised intracranial pressure may produce contralateral papilloedema (**Foster–Kennedy syndrome**).
- Occasionally, meningiomas may spread in a thin layer over the dural surface rather than forming a rounded mass ('**meningioma en plaque**'). These lesions may present with progressive cranial nerve palsies.

Acoustic neuroma

This benign tumour, better termed a **schwannoma**, arises from nerve sheath cells in the eighth nerve complex in the region of the internal auditory meatus. The typical initial presentation is with unilateral sensorineural hearing loss, caused by damage to the eighth nerve within the meatus (**intracanalicular lesion**). Subsequent expansion of the tumour into the **cerebellopontine angle** (Fig. 13.8) involves adjacent cranial nerves (V and VII). Further tumour growth produces ipsilateral ataxia as a result of brainstem–cerebellar com-

pression and lower (bulbar) cranial nerve palsies. Ultimately, features of raised intracranial pressure develop, especially when hydrocephalus supervenes because of obstruction at the level of the fourth ventricle. Other tumours may occasionally affect the cerebellopontine angle, including meningiomas and metastases.

Pituitary adenoma

When a pituitary tumour expands, it may involve structures above and on either side of the pituitary fossa (**suprasellar** and **parasellar** extension, respectively). The classical neurological manifestation of such a lesion is bitemporal hemianopia (Chapter 4), caused by compression of the optic chiasm by suprasellar extension of an adenoma (Fig. 13.9). Other pathological entities that may produce chiasmatic compression, mimicking a pituitary adenoma, include:

- carotid aneurysm,
- suprasellar meningioma,
- craniopharyngioma – a tumour arising from developmental cell rests of buccal epithelium close to the pituitary stalk in an embryological remnant (Rathke's pouch).

Pituitary adenomas present with endocrine disease in combination with or in the absence of visual field defects. Tumour cells may be functioning, i.e. secreting anterior pituitary hormones (acromegaly caused by growth hormone

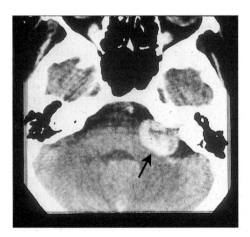

Figure 13.8 Acoustic neuroma (arrowed).

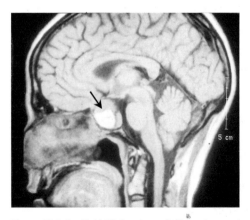

Figure 13.9 Sagittal MRI showing a pituitary adenoma (arrowed). The high signal is due to haemorrhage within the tumour.

excess, prolactinomas, Cushing's disease caused by corticotrophin-secreting tumours). Alternatively, patients may develop hypopituitarism because of suppression of normal cells in the gland by the tumour. Occasionally, pituitary adenomas undergo acute infarction. Patients may present with sudden headache and vomiting (resembling subarachnoid haemorrhage) and acute hypopituitarism (**pituitary apoplexy**). Swelling of necrotic tumour tissue produces rapidly evolving bitemporal hemianopia with bilateral ophthalmoplegia as a result of parasellar extension into the cavernous sinuses.

Visual field defects caused by pituitary adenomas typically first involve the superior temporal quadrants, as the chiasm is being compressed from below. Conversely, craniopharyngiomas tend to exert chiasmatic pressure from above, affecting the inferior temporal quadrants first. Craniopharyngiomas are also distinct from pituitary adenomas in their other neuroendocrine manifestations:

- growth failure in childhood (the tumours may present in childhood, adolescence or adult life),
- diabetes insipidus,
- obstructive hydrocephalus caused by expansion of the tumour into the third ventricle.

Other tumours and cysts

Rarer tumour syndromes include:
- colloid cysts – cystic tumours derived from embryological remnants in the third ventricle, which may produce acute obstructive hydrocephalus,
- tumours in the pineal region – which present with eye movement disorders, especially impaired upgaze caused by proximity of the lesion to the superior midbrain, and obstructive hydrocephalus at third ventricle level,
- haemangioblastoma – vascular tumour arising in the cerebellum and occasionally elsewhere,
- skull base tumours may extend intracranially, producing multiple cranial nerve palsies.

Management of brain tumours
Surgery

Benign tumours are often amenable to complete excision and surgery is potentially curative. For malignant primary or secondary tumours, cure is generally not possible.

Surgery for primary tumours is, however, often indicated to reach a histological diagnosis and, if possible, to alleviate symptoms by reducing tumour bulk. Histological examination of biopsies from presumed primary tumours serves to confirm that the lesion is a glioma and not another neoplasm, e.g. lymphoma, or even a non-neoplastic condition, e.g. abscess. It also permits **grading** of the degree of differentiation of the tumour, which correlates with prognosis. Thus, patients with grade 1–2 gliomas may survive many years. But the median survival for the most poorly differentiated tumours (grade 4) is 9 months.

Sometimes, surgery is not advisable, e.g., in patients with presumed low-grade gliomas presenting with epilepsy only. Surgery would also be inappropriate for multiple brain metastases, where the diagnosis is clear, though some solitary metastases are amenable to resection.

Radiotherapy

Gliomas may be treated by radiotherapy directed towards the tumour, whereas metastases are treated by whole-brain radiation. Radiotherapy is also used in the management of some benign tumours, e.g. pituitary adenomas.

Drug treatment

- Anti-epileptic drugs for epilepsy.
- Corticosteroids (dexamethasone) for raised intracranial pressure. Steroids may also temporarily improve focal neurological deficits by treating brain oedema.
- Chemotherapy – may be indicated in some patients with glioma, in addition to surgery and radiotherapy, under the supervision of specialized neuro-oncology units. Novel chemotherapeutic agents (such as temozolomide) and drug delivery systems (including directly into the tumour cavity) are available, but the prognosis for high-grade gliomas remains very poor.

Key points

- Raised intracranial pressure may prove fatal due to brainstem compression
- Rising intracranial pressure due to mass lesions may be exacerbated by hydrocephalus, if the normal flow of CSF is obstructed, and by cerebral oedema
- Admission to hospital after head injury is essential in the presence of a depressed conscious level, skull fracture or focal neurological signs
- Brain tumours may present with epilepsy, raised intracranial pressure or focal neurological deficits

Headache due to intracranial tumour

Case history: A 15-year-old boy developed daily occipital headaches which became progressively more severe over the course of 6 weeks. The pain was present on waking and would gradually clear later in the day. In the week leading up to presentation, the pain was very severe and he needed to stop, when walking to school, to vomit. Neurological examination was normal.

Comment: Despite the normal examination findings, this patient required immediate admission and investigation. His vomiting was not a manifestation of school refusal, as suggested by the referring doctor, but was highly suspicious of a posterior fossa mass. This was confirmed by urgent MRI, which showed a large cystic lesion in the left cerebellar hemisphere with distortion of the fourth ventricle and obstructive hydrocephalus. At operation, a cystic (pilocytic) cerebellar astrocytoma was excised. This is a relatively benign lesion, and resection is usually curative.

Chapter 14

Neurological infections

Bacterial (pyogenic) meningitis

Aetiology

In the developed world, most cases of bacterial meningitis are caused by infection of the meninges by:
- *Neisseria meningitidis* (meningococcus), or
- *Streptococcus pneumoniae* (pneumococcus).

Other organisms, importantly including *Mycobacterium tuberculosis*, may be found in specific at-risk groups, e.g. immunocompromised patients (Table 14.1). *Haemophilus influenzae* (type b) has become much rarer following the introduction of vaccine.

Epidemiology

The incidence of bacterial meningitis is 5–10 in 100,000 per annum in developed countries.

The two common organisms have particular patterns of occurrence:
- Meningococcal meningitis may occur in epidemics.
- Pneumococcal infection is more common in older patients and is also associated with

alcoholism and splenectomy. It may spread to the meninges from adjacent structures (ears, nasopharynx) or from the lungs by the bloodstream.

Clinical features

Headache is typically severe and may be associated with pain and stiffness in the neck and back, vomiting and photophobia. The speed of onset of headache is rapid (minutes to hours), though not usually as sudden as with subarachnoid haemorrhage (Chapter 11). Patients may present with an altered level of consciousness and seizures.

General examination reveals signs of infection, including fever, tachycardia, shock and sometimes evidence of the primary source of infection (e.g., pneumonia, endocarditis, sinusitis, otitis media). A rash is present in most patients with meningococcal meningitis, typically petechial or purpuric.

Neurological signs include:
- **'meningism'** – evidence of meningeal irritation – neck stiffness on attempted flexion, high-pitched 'meningeal cry' in infants, **Kernig's sign** (Chapter 9),
- deteriorating level of consciousness,
- raised intracranial pressure – papilloedema, bulging fontanelle in infants,
- cranial nerve palsies and other focal signs.

Lecture Notes: Neurology, 9th edition. By Lionel Ginsberg. Published 2010 by Blackwell Publishing.

Table 14.1 Rarer causes of bacterial meningitis in at-risk groups.

Enterobacteriaceae, group B streptococci – neonates
Listeria monocytogenes – neonates, immunocompromised patients
Mycobacterium tuberculosis – immunocompromised patients and those from developing countries
Staphylococci – patients with head injuries or neurosurgical shunts

Investigations and diagnosis

- **Lumbar puncture** in untreated acute bacterial meningitis reveals
  - turbid CSF,
  - raised CSF pressure,
  - polymorph leucocytosis (hundreds or thousands of cells per μL),
  - raised protein concentration (more than 1 g/L),
  - low glucose concentration (less than half blood concentration, but frequently undetectable).

  The causative organism may be identified on Gram stain or by culture or molecular techniques.
- Contraindications to lumbar puncture in patients with suspected meningitis include papilloedema, deteriorating level of consciousness and focal neurological signs. In such patients, pre-puncture cranial CT scan is needed to exclude a mass lesion, e.g. in the posterior fossa, which may mimic meningitis.
- Other investigations include
  - full blood count (neutrophilia),
  - coagulation studies (disseminated intravascular coagulation),
  - electrolytes (hyponatraemia),
  - blood cultures (may be positive even if CSF is sterile),
  - chest and skull (sinus) radiography (to identify primary source of infection).

Complications

Acute complications of meningitis include seizures, abscess formation, hydrocephalus, inappropriate antidiuretic hormone secretion and septic shock.

A particularly severe manifestation of septic shock with disseminated intravascular coagulation and adrenal haemorrhages is a complication of meningococcal meningitis (Waterhouse–Friderichsen syndrome). Meningococcal disease may also be complicated by arthritis, either directly septic or immune-complex mediated.

Management

- Bacterial meningitis may be fatal within hours: early diagnosis and treatment with high doses of appropriate intravenous antibiotics are essential.
- Benzylpenicillin is the drug of choice for meningococcal and pneumococcal infection if the prevalence of penicillin-resistant organisms is low. An initial dose of 2.4 g is followed by 1.2 g 2 hourly. Within 48–72 hours, if there is evidence of clinical improvement, the regimen can be relaxed to 4- or 6 hourly, though with the same total daily dose (14.4 g). Treatment should continue for 7 days after the patient has become afebrile (14 days for pneumococcus).
- Empirical antibiotic treatment where the prevalence of penicillin-resistant organisms exceeds 5% is generally with cefotaxime or ceftriaxone. Ampicillin should be added if the patient is immunosuppressed, pregnant or elderly (to cover *Listeria*). Vancomycin is indicated if there is a risk of *Staphylococcus aureus*, e.g. shunt-associated meningitis. Once the causative organism and antibiotic sensitivity are known, the patient should be changed to the appropriate medication.
- General practitioners should give patients with suspected meningococcal meningitis a single intravenous or intramuscular injection of benzylpenicillin before urgent admission to hospital.
- If lumbar puncture is delayed by the need for pre-puncture CT scan, antibiotic treatment should be started before the scan, after blood has been taken for culture.
- There is increasing evidence that initial treatment with high-dose intravenous corticosteroids (dexamethasone 0.4 mg/kg body weight daily for 4 days) in parallel with antibiotics improves

morbidity and mortality in bacterial meningitis, by reducing the inflammatory response.

• Other general treatment measures include bed rest, analgesics, antipyretics, anti-epilepsy drugs for seizures and supportive measures for coma, shock, raised intracranial pressure, electrolyte disturbances and bleeding disorders.

Prevention

• **Chemoprophylaxis** (rifampicin or ciprofloxacin) is indicated for household contacts in meningococcal meningitis.
• **Immunization** against *H. influenzae* infection (using *H. influenzae* type b vaccine) is recommended routinely for children at the ages of 2, 3 and 4 months, and has greatly reduced the incidence of meningitis caused by this organism.

Prognosis

The mortality from acute bacterial meningitis is approximately 10% overall – higher in *S. pneumoniae* infection.

Pneumococcal disease is also more likely to result in long-term sequelae (up to 30% of patients), including hydrocephalus, cranial nerve palsies, visual and motor deficits and epilepsy. Children with acute bacterial meningitis may be left with behavioural disturbances, learning difficulties, hearing loss and epilepsy.

Other bacterial infections

Brain abscess

Aetiology

Brain abscess is less common than bacterial meningitis but may complicate otitis media (giving rise particularly to temporal lobe and cerebellar abscess) and other local sites of infection (e.g., paranasal sinuses). It may also arise by distant spread from the lungs (bronchiectasis), pelvis or heart (bacterial endocarditis and congenital lesions).

Clinical features

A collection of pus produces predictable features of an expanding mass in the brain:
• raised intracranial pressure,
• focal signs (dysphasia, hemiparesis, ataxia),
• seizures.

Fever is common but does not always develop. The progression of symptoms and signs, typically over days or even a few weeks, may closely resemble that of a brain neoplasm.

Investigation

• CT scan or MRI is mandatory for suspected abscess (Fig. 14.1).
• Lumbar puncture is **contraindicated** (risk of coning – Chapter 13).
• Blood tests include full blood count (neutrophil leucocytosis) and blood cultures.

Management

• **Neurosurgical intervention** to decompress and drain the abscess may be necessary to treat the clinical features and achieve a bacteriological diagnosis.
• **Broad-spectrum antibiotics** (e.g., cefotaxime plus metronidazole) are required until an accurate bacteriological diagnosis has been reached.
• **Corticosteroids** (with antibiotic cover) may be required to treat cerebral oedema.

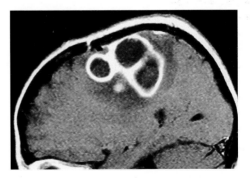

Figure 14.1 Parasagittal MRI showing a multilocular cerebral abscess. Note the central low signal, prominent 'ring enhancement' (high signal) (scanned after intravenous gadolinium) and surrounding oedema (low signal again).

Parameningeal infections

Pus may also accumulate in the epidural space, particularly in the spine. The causative organism is usually *S. aureus* from a distant skin infection. There may be osteomyelitis of the vertebrae and infection of intervertebral discs in association with a spinal epidural abscess. Patients present with severe back pain, fever (which may not be marked) and a rapidly evolving paraparesis. Investigation is by spinal MR imaging and blood cultures. Treatment is with anti-staphylococcal antibiotics and early surgical intervention if there is evidence of neural compression.

Local infections of the face and scalp may spread to the intracranial subdural space (**subdural empyema**) and to the intracranial venous sinuses, the latter resulting in septic venous sinus and cortical venous thrombosis (Chapter 11).

Tuberculosis

Tuberculous meningitis typically presents less acutely than purulent bacterial meningitis, and clinical diagnosis can be difficult. Immunocompromised individuals and those from ethnic minorities and immigrant populations are particularly at risk. Clinical features include persistent headache, fever, seizures and focal neurological signs, often developing over several weeks. The CSF is at raised pressure and may contain several hundred cells per microlitre (mixed polymorphs and lymphocytes), with raised protein and low glucose. Though organisms may be seen on auramine or Ziehl–Neelsen staining, they are frequently not found and bacteriological diagnosis may require multiple CSF specimens and CSF culture. Detection of mycobacterial nucleic acid by the polymerase chain reaction is an additional diagnostic technique. Treatment, however, should not be delayed in suspected cases, and is initially with isoniazid (with pyridoxine cover), rifampicin, pyrazinamide and a fourth drug, usually ethambutol or streptomycin. Antituberculous chemotherapy must be continued long term (9–12 months or more) and under the supervision of a tuberculosis specialist. The pyrazinamide and fourth drug may be discontinued after 2 months. Corticosteroids are used initially, in combination with antituberculous drugs, to suppress the host's inflammatory response and hence reduce the risk of cerebral oedema.

M. tuberculosis may also produce chronic caseating granulomas (**tuberculomas**), which act as intracranial mass lesions. These may arise during the course of tuberculous meningitis or as isolated phenomena. Spinal tuberculosis may result in cord compression (Pott's disease of the spine). Other complications of tuberculous meningitis include hydrocephalus and stroke-like events. The case fatality and morbidity of the disease remain high (both up to 30%) despite treatment.

Syphilis

Neurosyphilis is still seen, particularly among the homosexual population in the context of HIV (see below), though the parenchymatous forms of the disease are now rare. There are several distinct clinical entities:
- mild self-limiting meningitis of secondary syphilis,
- **meningovascular syphilis**: inflammation of meninges and cerebrospinal arteries in tertiary syphilis – presenting as subacute meningitis with focal signs, e.g. cranial nerve palsies, hemiparesis, paraparesis and wasting of the intrinsic hand muscles (**syphilitic amyotrophy**),
- **gumma** – focal meningovascular disease presenting as an intracranial mass lesion, e.g. with epilepsy, focal deficits, raised intracranial pressure,
- **tabes dorsalis** – parenchymatous disease primarily affecting dorsal root ganglion cells of spinal cord (Fig. 14.2),
- **'general paralysis of the insane'** – parenchymatous disease of the brain (Fig. 14.2),
- **congenital neurosyphilis**.

The diagnosis of neurosyphilis is reached by **serological tests for syphilis** in blood and CSF. The CSF may also show up to 100 lymphocytes/μL, raised protein and oligoclonal bands (Chapters 8 and 16). Treatment is with intramuscular procaine penicillin, 1.8–2.4 g daily for 17 days, in

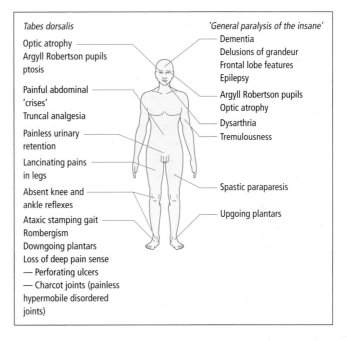

Tabes dorsalis	'General paralysis of the insane'

Optic atrophy
Argyll Robertson pupils
ptosis

Painful abdominal
'crises'
Truncal analgesia

Painless urinary
retention

Lancinating pains
in legs

Absent knee and
ankle reflexes

Ataxic stamping gait
Rombergism
Downgoing plantars
Loss of deep pain sense
— Perforating ulcers
— Charcot joints (painless
hypermobile disordered
joints)

Dementia
Delusions of grandeur
Frontal lobe features
Epilepsy

Argyll Robertson pupils
Optic atrophy

Dysarthria
Tremulousness

Spastic paraparesis

Upgoing plantars

Figure 14.2 Clinical features of neurosyphilis.

combination with oral probenecid. Steroid cover is advisable during initial penicillin therapy to avoid the **Jarisch–Herxheimer reaction** – an inflammatory response to the rapid killing of spirochaetes.

Lyme disease

Infection with the spirochaete *Borrelia burgdorferi*, which is transmitted by tick bite, may produce neurological manifestations in addition to the systemic features of the disease. In the acute phase, i.e. the first month after tick bite, meningism may occur, along with fever, rash and joint pains. Chronic disease, developing weeks or months after the bite, may be characterized neurologically by meningitis, encephalitis, cranial nerve palsies (especially the facial nerve), spinal root and peripheral nerve lesions. Serological tests may support the clinical diagnosis. The organism is usually sensitive to cefotaxime or ceftriaxone.

Leprosy

Mycobacterium leprae is one of the few micro-organisms that directly invade peripheral nerves.

Patients with 'tuberculoid leprosy', the more benign and less infectious form of the disease, have a patchy sensory polyneuropathy with palpable thickened nerves and depigmented anaesthetic areas of skin. Though the disease is very rare in Europe and North America, it is probably the most common cause of a multifocal neuropathy (Chapter 17) worldwide.

Bacterial toxins

Disease of the nervous system may arise from the action of toxins produced by certain bacteria.

● **Tetanus** toxin, from *Clostridium tetani* in wound infections, produces tonic spasms of the jaw ('lockjaw' – **trismus**) and trunk (**opisthotonos**), then fever with painful paroxysmal spasms of the whole body, with arched back, clenched teeth and extended limbs. Treatment in an intensive care unit involves muscle relaxants and ventilatory support, along with human antitetanus immunoglobulin, penicillin and wound cleansing. The disease would be eradicated if active immunization with **tetanus toxoid** was universally followed.

- **Botulism** is a consequence of toxin production by *Clostridium botulinum*, a contaminant in inadequately sterilized canned foods. The disease is also encountered in heroin addicts, in whom the organism may infect skin wounds. Patients with food botulism experience diarrhoea and vomiting and then develop paralysis within 2 days of toxin ingestion. The weakness is typically 'descending' in evolution – first ptosis, diplopia and paralysis of accommodation, then severe weakness of the bulbar and limb muscles. Assisted ventilation is generally required and recovery is very slow – months or even years.

- **Diphtheria** toxin may cause a polyneuropathy; fortunately, this condition is now very rare in developed countries with the advent of immunization.

Viral infections

Viral meningitis

Infection with mumps, enteroviruses and some other viruses may produce a benign self-limiting illness without the severe complications of acute bacterial meningitis. The CSF pressure may be raised and several hundred cells present per microlitre, though usually lymphocytes with few polymorphs except in the early stages of infection. Protein concentration may be modestly elevated, and glucose concentration is normal. The differential diagnosis of a patient presenting with meningism and a CSF lymphocytosis – the syndrome of **'aseptic meningitis'** – is broad (Table 14.2).

Viral encephalitis

Aetiology and pathogenesis

Viral invasion of the brain may produce a lymphocytic inflammatory reaction with necrosis of neurones and glia.

Herpes simplex virus type 1 is the most common cause of sporadic encephalitis in the developed world. Other viral causes include herpes zoster, cytomegalovirus, Epstein–Barr virus (all herpesviruses, particularly relevant in immuno-

Table 14.2 Differential diagnosis of aseptic meningitis.

Partially treated bacterial meningitis
Viral meningitis and meningoencephalitis
Tuberculous meningitis
Syphilis
Leptospirosis, brucellosis – in at-risk groups
Cerebral malaria
Fungal meningitis
Parameningeal infection – spinal or intracranial abscess, venous sinus thrombosis, occult paranasal sinus infection
Endocarditis
Malignant meningitis – carcinoma, lymphoma, leukaemia
Subarachnoid haemorrhage
Chemical meningitis – myelography, drugs
Sarcoidosis
Autoimmune disease, vasculitis, Behçet's disease
Mollaret's meningitis – recurrent fever, meningism and CSF lymphocytosis, probably associated with herpes virus infections

compromised patients), adenovirus and mumps. Encephalitis may occur in epidemics, as a result of arbovirus infection in parts of the world where mosquitoes act as vectors for these diseases.

Clinical features

Patients present with headache, fever and deteriorating level of consciousness over hours or days. Seizures may occur, and focal neurological signs may point to cerebral hemispheric or brainstem dysfunction. Hemispheric signs (dysphasia, hemiparesis) increase the likelihood of herpes simplex encephalitis.

Investigations

- CT scan and MRI of the brain may exclude mass lesions and show brain swelling. The characteristic appearances of herpes simplex encephalitis (Fig. 14.3) may take several days to develop.
- CSF is under increased pressure, usually with a lymphocytosis, raised protein and normal glucose. For diagnosing herpes simplex encephalitis, viral antibody titres are helpful only in retrospect. Early diagnosis may now be achieved with viral antigen

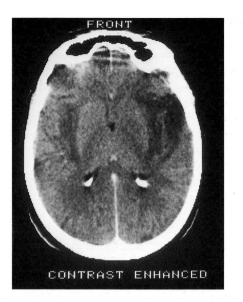

Figure 14.3 Herpes simplex encephalitis. Note the asymmetrical low density in the temporal lobes.

immunoassay and the polymerase chain reaction for amplification of viral DNA.
• EEG is abnormal with evidence of diffuse brain dysfunction. In herpes simplex encephalitis, characteristic **periodic complexes** may be present over the temporal region.

Management

Aciclovir (10 mg/kg intravenously every 8 hours for 14 days) has revolutionized the treatment of herpes simplex encephalitis, reducing mortality and morbidity. Death and serious disability (epilepsy, dysphasia and amnesic syndrome) still result, particularly when diagnosis and treatment are delayed. Thus, aciclovir should be started early if the diagnosis is suspected without waiting for results of detailed CSF studies and without brain biopsy, which is seldom warranted.

Specific treatment is not available for other causes of encephalitis, with the exception of a role for **ganciclovir** if cytomegalovirus infection is suspected. Patients, however, require supportive measures, including anti-epilepsy drugs for seizures and dexamethasone or mannitol for worsening cerebral oedema.

Herpes zoster

Varicella zoster virus, dormant in dorsal root ganglion cells after an initial chickenpox infection, may reactivate as shingles. The patient may experience localized pain and itching before the appearance of the characteristic unilateral vesicular rash, which affects a single dermatome or a few adjacent dermatomes, often on the trunk. After the rash has healed, pain may persist and prove difficult to treat (**post-herpetic neuralgia**, Chapter 9).

Variants include:
• **Zoster ophthalmicus** – where the rash involves the ophthalmic division of the trigeminal nerve, with a risk of corneal damage, and of troublesome facial post-herpetic neuralgia,
• **Ramsay Hunt syndrome** – with unilateral LMN facial palsy and vesicles in the external auditory meatus or on the fauces. There may be severe ear pain and occasionally associated vertigo, tinnitus and hearing loss (**zoster oticus**).
• **Motor zoster** – muscle weakness involving myotomes at a similar level to the dermatomes affected by the rash, e.g. unilateral diaphragmatic palsy in association with a rash on one side of the neck and one shoulder (C3, C4, C5 dermatomes).

Although shingles is usually a self-limiting illness, it warrants treatment with aciclovir, in higher oral doses than for superficial herpes simplex infections, to speed healing and reduce pain and the risk of complications.

Zoster infection may produce more severe manifestations, particularly in immunocompromised individuals, including a generalized rash, and encephalitis. Some patients have selective involvement of the spinal cord (zoster myelitis) or of cerebral vessels, which may present as hemiplegia.

Retroviral infections

Infection with human immunodeficiency virus, HIV, may lead to neurological complications for two reasons. First, the virus itself has an affinity for neural tissue, i.e. it is neurotropic as well as lymphotropic. Thus, a meningitic illness may occur at seroconversion. Later, a slowly progressive dementia and involvement of other parts of the nervous system, particularly the spinal cord and peripheral nerves, may develop. The second reason for neurological disease is the risk of opportunistic infection and unusual neoplasms involving the nervous system as a result of immunocompromise in full-blown AIDS.

• **Cerebral toxoplasmosis** – the presence of focal hemispheric (hemiparesis, dysphasia, extrapyramidal disorders), cerebellar (ataxia) or cranial nerve deficits in an AIDS patient, possibly with headache and seizures, and with CT or MRI evidence of focal or multifocal encephalitis warrants anti-toxoplasma treatment with pyrimethamine, folinic acid and either sulphadiazine or clindamycin. Brain biopsy is generally reserved for non-responders to this treatment.

• **Cryptococcal meningitis** – the yeast *Cryptococcus neoformans* is the most common cause of meningitis in AIDS patients. The clinical presentation is with acute or subacute headache, fever and sometimes seizures and focal neurological deficits. CSF examination (after CT scan to exclude intracranial mass lesion) reveals a lymphocytosis, usually with raised protein and low glucose. Cryptococci may be identified on an Indian ink preparation or by detection of antigen in CSF or blood. Treatment is with combined antifungal drugs (amphotericin B and flucytosine), though this may be unsuccessful. Cryptococcal meningitis may complicate other immunosuppressed states, e.g. post-organ transplantation.

• **Herpesviruses** – cytomegalovirus infection is common in AIDS patients and may result in encephalitis or cord involvement. Other herpesviruses, e.g. herpes simplex and herpes zoster, may also produce focal or diffuse encephalitis.

• **Progressive multifocal leucoencephalopathy** (**PML**) is due to opportunistic infection by papovaviruses (JC and others), resulting in multiple white matter lesions in the cerebral hemispheres, brainstem and cerebellum, presenting with progressive dementia and focal deficits, e.g. hemiparesis and dysphasia. Death is usual within months. PML may occur in other immunodeficiency states, e.g. haematological malignancies, tuberculosis, sarcoidosis.

• **Cerebral lymphoma** may present with focal or multifocal disease in the cerebral hemispheres and posterior fossa, both clinically and on CT or MR imaging. The diagnosis may be made on brain biopsy in non-responders to anti-toxoplasma therapy.

All these complications have become less common in developed countries with the advent of highly active antiretroviral therapy (HAART).

Retroviruses other than HIV are also neurotropic. Thus, the virus HTLV-1, prevalent in certain areas, e.g. the Caribbean, is associated with **tropical spastic paraparesis** (HTLV-1-associated myelopathy, HAM).

Other viruses

• **Poliomyelitis** is now rare in developed countries following the uptake of immunization. In previous epidemics, most patients experienced only the 'minor illness' characterized by headache, fever and vomiting 7–14 days after the virus entered the body through the gut or nasopharynx. Some, however, went on to a preparalytic stage as the virus gained access to the CNS, with meningitis, spinal and limb pain. Because of the virus' tropism for the anterior horn cells of the spinal cord and equivalent cells in the brainstem, a further proportion developed the paralytic illness with progressive muscle weakness over several days. Clinical features are exclusively those of LMN damage, with variable, often patchy and asymmetrical muscle involvement, fasciculation in the early stages and later wasting and areflexia. Only a minority of patients develop bulbar and respiratory failure. Though some recovery occurs at the end of the paralytic stage, many patients are left with permanent weakness and a few require long-term ventilatory support. The **post-polio syndrome** is a controversial entity, late deterioration in poliomyelitis victims generally being due to the superadded effects of other illnesses.

• **Rabies** has been eradicated from the UK and several other countries but remains endemic elsewhere. The disease is usually acquired by the bite of an infected dog, but it may be transmitted by other mammals. The virus migrates slowly (days or weeks) from the site of the bite to the CNS, where it excites an inflammatory reaction, with diagnostic intracytoplasmic inclusions (**Negri bodies**) seen within neurones *post-mortem*. If the brunt of the inflammatory change is in the brainstem, 'furious' rabies develops after a prodrome of fever and psychiatric disorder. Patients experience laryngospasm and terror on attempting to drink – **hydrophobia**. If the inflammation predominantly involves the spinal cord, there is a flaccid paralysis – 'dumb' or 'paralytic' rabies. Rabies is almost invariably fatal, once symptoms are established. Prophylactic immunization is available for those handling potentially infected animals, and active and passive immunization should be commenced immediately after a bite from such an animal, along with thorough wound cleansing.

Postviral phenomena

• **Subacute sclerosing panencephalitis** is a late and virtually universally fatal complication of measles infection, fortunately now very rare, particularly with the availability of immunization.
• **Acute disseminated encephalomyelitis** is a rare sequel of viral infection (Chapter 16).
• **Guillain–Barré syndrome** is associated with antecedent infection, often viral, in most patients (Chapter 20).
• Other neurological and psychiatric symptoms, particularly fatigue and impaired concentration and memory, may complicate recovery from virus infections, particularly the Epstein–Barr virus – **postviral fatigue syndrome** (Chapter 19).

Other infections and transmissible disorders

Protozoa

• **Malaria** must be considered, and formally excluded on blood films, in febrile individuals returning from endemic areas. *Plasmodium falciparum* infection causes a haemorrhagic encephalitis.
• **Toxoplasmosis** has been mentioned as a cause of multifocal encephalitis in AIDS patients, but it may also be acquired *in utero*, leading to hydrocephalus, intracranial calcification and choroidoretinitis.
• **Trypanosomiasis** in tropical Africa presents as a low-grade encephalitis, with hypersomnolence and seizures ('sleeping sickness').

Metazoa

Encysted tapeworm larvae may present as cerebral lesions.
• In **hydatid disease**, cysts may act as intracranial masses but rupture may result in chemical meningitis.
• In **cysticercosis**, the presence of multiple cysts may lead to epilepsy, raised intracranial pressure, focal neurological signs or hydrocephalus. Treatment is with praziquantel and steroid cover.

Prion disorders

These are considered in Chapter 18.

Key points

• Bacterial meningitis may prove fatal within hours
• General practitioners should give patients with suspected meningococcal meningitis a single parenteral dose of benzylpenicillin before urgent transfer to hospital
• Tuberculous meningitis should be suspected in at-risk individuals (immunocompromised patients or those from ethnic minorities and immigrant populations)
• 'Aseptic meningitis' has many causes – both infective and non-infective
• Neurological complications of HIV infection may be due to the virus itself, or to opportunistic infections resulting from immunocompromise in AIDS

Pyogenic (acute bacterial) meningitis

Case history: A 56-year-old man was brought unconscious to the casualty department of a district hospital. No antecedent history was available. On examination, he was pyrexial, 38.5°C, with neck stiffness but no other focal neurological signs; Glasgow Coma Scale was 6. A presumptive diagnosis of pyogenic meningitis was made, but the admitting physician rightly wanted the patient to undergo CT scanning before lumbar puncture, in view of the altered level of consciousness. No CT scanner was available out of hours at the district hospital, so the regional neurological centre was contacted.

The correct management advice given by the duty neurologist was for the patient immediately to receive high-dose intravenous antibiotics (benzylpenicillin and cefotaxime) at the local hospital, before transfer, once blood cultures had been taken. Following transfer, a CT cranial scan was normal and lumbar puncture yielded turbid CSF with 2000 polymorphs/μL, protein concentration 2.8 g/L, glucose undetectable. No organisms were seen on Gram stain and no bacteria were cultured from the CSF, but meningococci were grown from the blood cultures. The organism was fully sensitive to penicillin which was continued intravenously in anti-meningitic doses, and the patient made a full recovery.

Comment: Meningococcal meningitis typically occurs in childhood or adolescence, but can affect any age group, and a rash need not be present. Delayed treatment of pyogenic meningitis is associated with high mortality and morbidity. Pre-puncture CT scan is indicated in a patient with altered level of consciousness, but the potential delay in this patient's case necessitated pre-emptive antibiotic therapy. Though this sterilized the CSF, the diagnosis was reached by alternative means.

Herpes simplex encephalitis

Case history: A 47-year-old accountant developed a worsening headache over the course of 4 days. By the fourth day, he was nauseated and had vomited. His family brought him to hospital the next day saying he had become confused and was experiencing visual hallucinations. On admission, his temperature was 38.3°C. He was mildly dysphasic with word-finding difficulties. There were no focal signs in cranial nerve territory or the limbs. Tendon reflexes were symmetrical with downgoing plantar responses. He suffered a generalized seizure in the casualty department. CT cranial scan showed low density in the temporal lobes, worse on the left (see Fig. 14.3). An EEG revealed high-voltage slow waves in the left frontotemporal region but no epileptiform discharges. CSF examination was abnormal with 165 mononuclear cells/μL, no polymorphs or red cells. CSF protein was mildly elevated, but glucose was normal. Herpes simplex virus DNA was subsequently detected in the CSF by polymerase chain reaction amplification. Intravenous aciclovir was started on the day of admission at a dose of 10 mg/kg 8 hourly for 14 days along with supportive measures, including anti-epilepsy medication. He recovered but was left with persistently impaired recent verbal memory and mild word-finding difficulty. He was unable to return to his previous occupation.

Comment: The acute presentation with headache, fever, dysphasia and a seizure is highly suggestive of herpes simplex encephalitis. This diagnosis was supported by the characteristic CT changes, slow waves on EEG (not all patients develop periodic complexes), lymphocytic CSF and ultimately demonstration of viral DNA in the CSF. Treatment with antiviral medication should not be delayed while waiting for investigation results. Despite the improvements in mortality and morbidity achieved following the introduction of aciclovir, many patients are still left with persistent cognitive deficits, as in this example.

Chapter 15

Spinal conditions

Spinal cord disease (myelopathy)

Clinical neuroanatomy

Figure 15.1 is a transverse section of the spinal cord, showing the location of the major tracts. The main motor pathway, the corticospinal tract, is largely crossed, the UMNs having originated in the contralateral cerebral cortex. Similarly, the spinothalamic tract is crossed, conveying sensory information from the opposite side of the body, whereas the posterior columns convey ipsilateral information concerning position and vibration sense.

Symptoms and signs

Because of the proximity of the many nerve pathways in the cord, patients often present with simultaneous motor, sensory and autonomic dysfunction.

Motor

Typically patients have symptoms and signs of UMN damage affecting both legs (**spastic paraparesis**) or, if the lesion is in the high cervi-

Lecture Notes: Neurology, 9th edition. By Lionel Ginsberg. Published 2010 by Blackwell Publishing.

cal cord, all four limbs (**spastic tetraparesis**). Cervical cord lesions may alternatively produce a spastic paraparesis in combination with a mixture of LMN and UMN features in the upper limbs, because of simultaneous damage to the cord and to roots in the neck.

Sensory

The clinical hallmark of a spinal cord lesion is the presence of a **sensory level**, e.g. on the patient's trunk, below which cutaneous sensation is impaired and above which it returns to normal (see Fig. 6.1d). Though a sensory level in a patient with a spastic paraparesis is useful in confirming spinal cord pathology, it is of only limited value in anatomical localization. Thus, a level at T10 does not necessarily imply a cord lesion at T10 but rather that the lesion is at *or above* T10. This has important practical consequences. For example, a patient may present with clinical features of acute spinal cord compression, requiring urgent treatment. With a sensory level at T10, restricting imaging of the cord to the low thoracic region may result in a surgically treatable lesion further up being missed.

Autonomic

Bladder involvement is an early feature of spinal cord disease, patients complaining of urinary urgency and frequency, and eventually urge

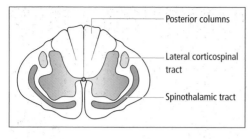

Figure 15.1 Transverse section of the spinal cord.

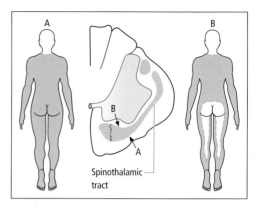

Figure 15.2 Extrinsic vs. intrinsic spinal cord lesions. In this section of part of the cervical cord, the lamination of the spinothalamic tract is indicated, fibres from the sacral dermatomes (S) outermost, then lumbar (L), then thoracic (T) and finally, most centrally, cervical (C). Extrinsic compression (A) involves the sacral dermatomes, whereas an intrinsic lesion (B) may result in sacral sparing.

incontinence of urine (Chapter 7). Bowel symptoms are less likely to develop early, though patients may complain of constipation. Sexual dysfunction, particularly erectile impotence, is common.

Other features of spinal cord disease include a history of neck or back pain or injury.

Specific cord syndromes

Extrinsic vs. intrinsic lesions

Extrinsic compression of the spinal cord, e.g. by tumour or prolapsed intervertebral disc, typically produces a pattern of sensory loss in which the sacral dermatomes are involved (**saddle anaesthesia**). This is because the part of the spinothalamic tract closest to the surface of the cord (that conveying sensory information from the lumbosacral dermatomes) is most vulnerable to the effects of external compression (Fig. 15.2). By contrast, intrinsic lesions of the spinal cord tend to damage the more central parts of the spinothalamic tract first (**sacral sparing**), though this is by no means a strict rule (Fig. 15.2).

Brown-Séquard syndrome

A characteristic pattern of sensory and motor deficits develops when a lesion damages only one side of the spinal cord. In its most complete form, caused by cord hemisection, this is termed a Brown-Séquard syndrome (Fig. 15.3). This syndrome is one situation where a sensory level does provide accurate localizing information.

Syringomyelia

This rare condition, in which a CSF-filled cavity (**syrinx**) develops centrally in the spinal cord (Fig. 15.4), also produces characteristic motor and sensory deficits (Fig. 15.5). Typically, the syrinx first evolves in the lower cervical cord (though over many years it may expand to occupy most of the cord). Patients, therefore, develop a spastic paraparesis but have LMN signs in the upper limbs (because of damage to both the corticospinal tracts and the anterior horns in the cervical cord). Posterior column function is relatively spared (**dissociated anaesthesia**), but spinothalamic sensation is severely affected as a result of interruption of the decussating pathways by the syrinx. The cutaneous loss (to pain and temperature sensation) is typically described as a 'cape' distribution or **suspended** sensory disturbance, with upper and lower levels determined by the extent of the syrinx. In some patients, the syrinx may extend into the medulla (**syringobulbia**) with the development of bilateral lower cranial nerve palsies and Horner's syndrome.

The pathogenesis of syringomyelia is poorly understood but is likely to involve abnormal CSF hydrodynamics. Many patients have an associated

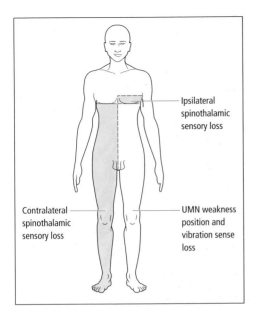

Figure 15.3 Brown-Séquard syndrome. There is UMN weakness on the same side as the lesion (as the descending corticospinal tracts have already crossed in the medulla). Position and vibration sensory loss are also ipsilateral to the lesion (as the ascending fibres in the posterior columns do not cross until they reach the medulla). Spinothalamic (pain and temperature) sensory loss is, however, contralateral to the lesion (as this pathway crosses the spinal cord at or just above its entry level). Patients may also have a narrow band of ipsilateral spinothalamic sensory loss (and sometimes pain) close to the level of the lesion, due to damage to the fibres which have not yet decussated to join the contralateral spinothalamic tract.

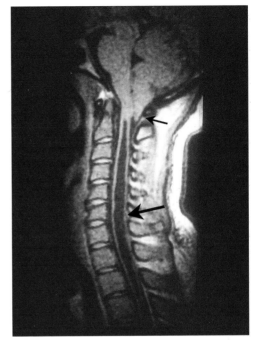

Figure 15.4 Syringomyelia. Sagittal MRI of the cervical spinal cord showing the fluid-filled syrinx cavity (low signal – large arrow) and associated Arnold–Chiari malformation (small arrow).

developmental abnormality of the brainstem and cerebellum (Arnold–Chiari malformation) in which the cerebellar tonsils are elongated and protrude through the foramen magnum (**cerebellar ectopia**). Thus, foramen magnum decompression has been advocated as surgical treatment for syringomyelia, as has drainage of the syrinx via a syringostomy.

If not developmental in origin, a syrinx may arise following trauma, or in association with a tumour of the spinal cord.

Other specific syndromes

Other 'classical' disturbances of spinal cord function, as a result of neurosyphilis (tabes dorsalis) and vitamin B_{12} deficiency (subacute combined degeneration of the cord), are described in Chapters 14 and 19, respectively. Spinal cord infarction caused by thrombosis of the anterior spinal artery typically spares posterior column function.

Causes of spinal cord disease

In patients aged 50+, the most common cause of myelopathy is **cervical spondylosis**. Here, degenerative disease (osteoarthritis) of the cervical spine may lead to cord compression with contributions from:

• calcification, degeneration and protrusion of intervertebral discs,
• bony outgrowths (**osteophytes**),
• calcification and thickening of longitudinal ligaments.

In patients aged 40 and under, multiple sclerosis is the most common explanation for a myelopathy sacral dermatomes (saddle anaesthesia). Anal tone is reduced and the anal reflex absent (S3/4/5 root value). This reflex is elicited by scratching the skin close to the anus – reflex sphincter constriction normally occurs. Urgent decompressive laminectomy is required after imaging has confirmed the diagnosis, to prevent irreversible sphincter dysfunction.

Key points

- Clinical features of spinal cord disease include a spastic paraparesis, sensory level and sphincter disturbance
- In older patients, spinal cord disease is commonly due to cervical spondylosis, whereas in younger patients, multiple sclerosis is the most common cause
- The most important aspect of the management of spinal cord disease is exclusion or detection of cord compression (by MR imaging or myelography)
- Patients with a prolapsed lumbar intervertebral disc typically present with sciatica and root tension signs (e.g., limited straight leg raising)
- Patients presenting acutely with bilateral sciatica and sphincter involvement require urgent imaging to detect a central disc prolapse compressing the cauda equina. If such a lesion is found, emergency decompressive surgery is essential to preserve sphincter function

---

Spinal cord compression

Case history: A 78-year-old man was admitted to hospital having become unable to walk during the previous 48 hours. His legs felt numb and he had been incontinent of urine. There was no spinal pain. On detailed questioning, he had been aware of mild but increasing difficulty walking and urgency of micturition over the previous 6 weeks, but had otherwise been well in the past. On examination, cranial nerves and upper limbs were normal. In the lower limbs, there was an increase in tone, with a pyramidal distribution of weakness in both legs. Knee and ankle reflexes were brisk with bilateral upgoing plantar responses. Position and vibration sense were impaired in the feet, and there was a sensory level to pinprick and light touch at T12. The admitting team organized immediate spinal MR imaging, directed towards the lumbar and lower thoracic spine, which was normal. The patient was therefore referred to the neurologists, on the assumption that a compressive spinal lesion had been excluded. Repeat MRI scanning of the whole spine revealed an epidural mass compressing the spinal cord at the cervicothoracic junction. The patient's prostate-specific antigen (PSA) was grossly elevated. He was referred to the oncologists and radiotherapists for appropriate immediate management of cord compression due to metastatic carcinoma of the prostate.

Comment: The combination of the UMN lower limb signs, bladder involvement and a sensory level clearly point to a spinal cord lesion. The admitting team's mistake was to assume that the T12 sensory level meant that the lesion was at that level, whereas in fact it was much higher. Acute spinal cord compression is an emergency requiring urgent decompressive treatment – neurosurgical or radiotherapeutic depending on the cause. Spinal pain is not a consistent clinical feature, though its presence may aid lesion localization.

Chapter 16

Multiple sclerosis

Multiple sclerosis (MS) is a disorder which, in its most typical form, is characterized by lesions separated both in space and time in the CNS. It is one of the most common chronic neurological conditions affecting young people.

Pathology and pathophysiology

The disease primarily affects the white matter of the brain and spinal cord, and the optic nerves. Chronic inflammatory cells are present and myelin is damaged, with relative sparing of axons, at least initially. These changes are not uniformly distributed. There are relatively normal-appearing regions of white matter interspersed with foci of inflammation and demyelination known as **plaques**, which are often located near venules. **Inflammatory demyelination** of CNS tracts leads to a reduction in their conduction velocity with distortion and ultimately loss of information conveyed by impulse traffic along these pathways.

Plaques evolve with time. At an early stage there is local breakdown of the blood–brain barrier, then evidence of inflammation with oedema, loss of myelin and eventually the CNS equivalent of scar tissue, **gliosis**. The final result, a shrunken area of sclerosis, may be associated with little clinical deficit compared with that

present when the plaque was pathologically most active. This is partly because of remyelination, for which the CNS has some potential, and also signifies a return of function with resolution of the inflammation and oedema. This pathological sequence corresponds to the clinical pattern of MS relapses, with symptoms being present for a period then resolving partially or completely. Further inflammatory lesions, close to sites of pre-existing damage, may contribute to the eventual accumulation of neurological deficit, but axonal loss, with consequent brain, cord and optic atrophy, is now recognized as a major pathological substrate for the progressive phase of the illness (see below). Plaques need not invariably be associated with specific clinical events, e.g. if they are small or occur in relatively 'silent' areas of the CNS.

Aetiology and pathogenesis

Uniting many strands of circumstantial evidence, a working hypothesis for the causation of MS is that an environmental agent, e.g. a virus, triggers the condition in a genetically susceptible individual.

The role of immune mechanisms in MS pathogenesis is supported by several findings, including the presence of chronic inflammatory cells in active plaques and linkage of the condition to specific genes in the major

Lecture Notes: Neurology, 9th edition. By Lionel Ginsberg. Published 2010 by Blackwell Publishing.

histocompatibility complex (MHC). Many 'autoimmune' disorders show linkage to this group of genes.

MHC linkage is also one of the lines of evidence for a genetic component in the aetiology of MS, as is the occurrence of familial cases, and the finding of increased concordance for the condition in identical (monozygous) as opposed to non-identical (dizygous) twins. However, no single gene has been shown to be necessary or sufficient for the development of MS.

Epidemiology

MS is more common in areas of temperate than tropical climate. Ethnic differences in incidence have been used as an argument in favour of genetic susceptibility to the condition. But the geographical variation may also suggest a role for environmental factors, e.g. viruses. This is particularly indicated by the suggested occurrence of MS 'epidemics', e.g. in the Faroe Islands and Iceland. There is also evidence that individuals born in an area of high risk for MS will carry that risk if they emigrate to an area of lower risk and vice versa, but only if migration occurs after the mid-teens. This implies that the hypothetical virus is acting in the first decade or two of life.

The disease is more common in females than males (approximately 3:1). It may develop at any age, though its first onset is rare in children and the elderly. The usual age of presentation is between 20 and 40 years. In the UK, its prevalence is approximately 1 in 1000.

Clinical features

Presentation

Common modes of presentation of MS include:
- visual disturbance,
- limb weakness,
- sensory disturbance.

Visual disturbance

Optic (retrobulbar) neuritis is a characteristic visual disturbance that may herald the onset of MS. The underlying pathology is inflammatory demyelination of one or (less commonly) both optic nerves. Symptoms of unilateral optic neuritis include:
- pain around one eye, particularly on eye movement;
- blurred vision, which may proceed to complete monocular blindness within days or weeks;
- loss of colour vision.

Examination may reveal, in addition to impaired visual acuity and colour vision:
- pink, swollen optic disc on fundoscopy – if the area of inflammatory demyelination is immediately behind the optic nerve head,
- visual field defect – typically a central scotoma in the affected eye,
- relative afferent pupillary defect (Chapter 4).

A bout of optic neuritis will usually resolve over a period of weeks or months, though the patient may be left with some impairment of vision in the affected eye, and fundoscopy will generally reveal optic disc pallor caused by optic atrophy. Optic disc swelling in the acute phase, if bilateral, must be distinguished from papilloedema caused by raised intracranial pressure, though they may look similar through the ophthalmoscope. In the latter, visual acuity is relatively much better preserved, and the only field defect in early papilloedema is enlargement of the physiological blind spot. An episode of optic neuritis does not necessarily signify that the patient will subsequently develop MS – it may be a monophasic illness, particularly in children and if bilateral.

Other visual disturbances at the onset of MS include diplopia, often associated with vertigo and nausea, hence indicative of a brainstem plaque. Examination in these circumstances may reveal an internuclear ophthalmoplegia (Chapter 4). There may be associated cerebellar ataxia.

Sensorimotor disturbances

Sensory and motor presentations generally imply a lesion in the spinal cord or cerebral hemispheres. For example, the patient may present with an asymmetrical spastic paraparesis and/or paraesthesiae, thermal anaesthesia and dysaesthesiae in the limbs. A lesion in the posterior columns of the cervical spinal cord may produce the near-pathognomonic symptom of rapid tingling sensations shooting down the arms or legs on neck flexion (**Lhermitte phenomenon**). In some patients, motor, sensory or indeed visual symptoms are temporarily much worse after a hot bath (**Uhthoff phenomenon**).

Other presentations

Pain is a less common symptom in MS, though some patients may experience typical trigeminal neuralgia as a result of a brainstem plaque and others may have pain in the limbs. There is an increased incidence of epilepsy in patients with MS. Some patients may present with bladder disturbance (urgency of micturition or urinary retention) and impotence.

Course

The usual temporal pattern of symptom evolution in a patient presenting in one of the above ways is that clinical features worsen over days or weeks, reach a plateau and then gradually resolve, partially or completely, over weeks or months. There may then be recurrences at unpredictable intervals, affecting the same or different parts of the CNS. The role of factors such as physical injury, intercurrent infection, pregnancy and emotional stress in precipitating a relapse is controversial.

Particularly with initial episodes there may be complete or near-complete symptomatic resolution (**relapsing–remitting disease**, approximately 70–80% of patients). However, subsequent episodes of demyelination may leave some residual disability, the patient eventually entering a secondary phase of steady progression without resolution (**secondary progressive disease**). Some patients (approximately 10–20%), particularly those presenting in middle life with a spastic paraparesis, will have no clear-cut relapses and remissions (**primary progressive disease**) (Fig. 16.1).

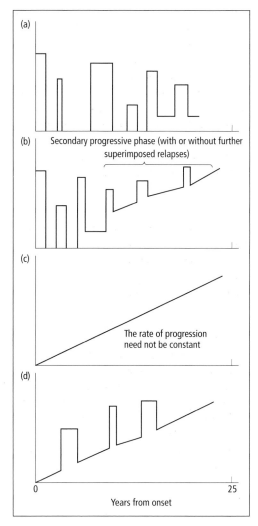

Figure 16.1 Clinical categories of MS: (a) relapsing–remitting; (b) secondary progressive (i.e., in a patient who previously had relapsing–remitting disease); (c) primary progressive; (d) progressive relapsing (rare).

The natural history of MS in individual patients is very variable. Some patients may have one or more initial episodes and then no symptoms for many years (10% follow this benign course). Others may accumulate disability, though remain able to work for years. However, a significant proportion of patients (up to one-third) are more severely affected. It is currently not possible to predict these individuals at onset, though that they may have experienced a 'one-off' illness. Patients may benefit from reading about MS or from contact with a local support society. However, the physician has a continuing educative role, particularly in guiding the patient with regard to potentially expensive treatments of unproven benefit, e.g. dietary manipulation and the use of hyperbaric oxygen.

While no cure is yet available for MS, there are three important aspects of treatment:

- management of an acute relapse,
- modification of the course of the disease,
- control of symptoms.

Management of an acute relapse

Individual relapses that are severe enough to limit function, e.g. because of limb weakness or visual failure, may be treated with corticosteroids. Currently, these are given in the form of high-dose methylprednisolone, intravenously or orally (500 mg to 1 g daily for 3–5 days). Such measures may improve the speed but not the degree of recovery from exacerbations. Longer-term steroids have not been shown to affect the natural history of the condition. It is advisable to exclude urinary tract infection before starting a course of corticosteroids.

Modification of the course of the disease

The evidence for an autoimmune basis for MS has prompted trials of immunosuppressant drugs, e.g. azathioprine, methotrexate and cyclophosphamide, in an effort to alter its long-term prognosis. However, any marginal benefit from these drugs is outweighed by side effects. More novel immunotherapeutic agents with the aim of altering the rate of progression of MS, or at least reducing relapse rate, without severe side effects, e.g. interferon-beta and glatiramer acetate, have now been introduced. These provide some protection against relapses (approximately 30% reduction in relapse frequency) and possibly a small slowing of the rate of progression. A monoclonal antibody, natalizumab, is approximately twice as effective as interferon-beta, and is used to treat aggressive relapsing–remitting MS. It has the drawback of a low risk of progressive multifocal leucoencephalopathy (Chapter 14). Mitoxantrone, a chemotherapeutic agent, is an alternative to natalizumab, but also has potentially serious adverse effects, including cardiotoxicity and a risk (0.2%) of acute leukaemia. Patients receiving any of these disease-modifying therapies are best managed in specialist MS clinics.

Control of symptoms

Symptomatic drug treatments for complications of MS are available as follows:

- Spasticity, flexor spasms – baclofen (oral or intrathecal), dantrolene, tizanidine, diazepam, though these drugs may increase weakness and cause drowsiness. Other approaches include botulinum toxin injections into affected muscles.
- Cerebellar tremor – if mild may respond to clonazepam, isoniazid or gabapentin.
- Fatigue (a common accompaniment of relapses) – amantadine, selegiline or the anti-narcolepsy drug modafinil.
- Bladder disturbances – anticholinergic drugs, e.g. oxybutynin or tolterodine; patients may also need to be taught intermittent self-catheterization (if post-micturition bladder residual volume exceeds 100 mL). Urinary infection should be treated promptly.
- Depression – tricyclic and related drugs in low dosage, e.g. amitriptyline or dosulepin; selective serotonin reuptake inhibitors, e.g. sertraline.
- Erectile impotence – phosphodiesterase type 5 inhibitors, e.g. sildenafil; intracavernosal papaverine or prostaglandins, the latter may also be given by urethral application.
- Pain, paroxysmal symptoms including seizures – carbamazepine, gabapentin. The role of cannabis in the management of pain and spasticity in MS is controversial.

Patients with more advanced MS may require the involvement of members of the neuro-rehabilitation team (Chapter 21). Severely affected patients need general measures appropriate to paraplegic patients, in particular careful nursing attention to pressure areas. Worsening urinary difficulty may necessitate urethral or suprapubic catheterization.

Other surgical measures in extreme instances include:

- tenotomy for spasticity and flexor spasms,
- dorsal column stimulation for pain,
- stereotactic thalamotomy for severe cerebellar ataxia.

Other diseases of myelin

Myelin is a target for various genetic and acquired diseases which are generally rarer than MS but enter its differential diagnosis.

Inherited disorders

Genetic disorders of myelin chemistry lead to abnormal myelin formation (**dysmyelination** rather than demyelination). These diseases, also known as the **leucodystrophies**, usually present in infancy or childhood. However, some develop in adulthood with dementia, ataxia, spasticity, seizures, optic atrophy and sometimes peripheral nervous system involvement (polyneuropathy). The disorders, fortunately all very rare, are progressive and fatal. No specific treatment is at present available, though there is interest in enzyme replacement by bone marrow transplantation or ultimately gene therapy.

Acquired disease

Acute disseminated encephalomyelitis (ADEM)

This is a rare disease characterized pathologically by acute multifocal inflammatory demyelination throughout the CNS. It may follow viral infection or immunization, hence it is also known as **postinfectious encephalomyelitis**.

Clinically, patients typically develop fever, headache and meningism. There may be impairment of consciousness and focal neurological symptoms and signs involving cerebral hemispheres, brainstem, cerebellum, spinal cord and optic nerves. Patients with postinfectious bilateral optic neuritis or isolated cord involvement (**transverse myelitis**) probably represent localized variants of ADEM.

Investigation reveals a CSF lymphocytosis (often several hundred cells) and raised protein. EEG changes are non-specific, and imaging by CT may be normal. MR imaging may show appearances similar to MS.

The differential diagnosis is with acute viral encephalitis (infectious rather than postinfectious, Chapter 14) and an acute attack of MS. Distinguishing ADEM from an attack of an illness that subsequently declares itself as MS may be difficult, but the presence of headache, fever, meningism, altered level of consciousness and high CSF lymphocyte count favour the former.

Treatment is with corticosteroids, usually high-dose intravenous methylprednisolone. Although a minority of patients die in the acute phase, the long-term prognosis in many is good, with complete recovery and no relapse.

Neuromyelitis optica (Devic's disease)

This is characterized by optic neuritis (unilateral or more typically bilateral) and transverse myelitis (see comment on case history at end of chapter).

Central pontine myelinolysis

This condition, which is associated with alcoholism and with hyponatraemia (and its over-rapid correction), presents acutely (over several days) with features of a pontine and medullary lesion, i.e. bulbar palsy, tetraparesis and subsequently eye movement disorder and coma. Treatment includes gradual correction of metabolic abnormalities, and vitamin supplements, though prognosis is poor.

Progressive multifocal leucoencephalopathy

This is considered in Chapter 14.

Key points

Multiple sclerosis:
- is characterized by two or more lesions in the CNS, separated in both space and time
- is the most common cause of chronic neurological disability in young people in developed countries
- is recognized pathologically by plaques of inflammatory demyelination
- may present with visual disturbance, sensory disturbance or limb weakness
- may have a relapsing–remitting or progressive course
- relapses may be treated with high-dose methylprednisolone if the episode is functionally limiting
- may potentially have its natural history altered by novel immunotherapeutic agents, e.g. interferon-beta

Multiple sclerosis

Case history: A 22-year-old woman developed loss of vision on the left over 48 hours, with pain around the left eye on eye movement. At her worst, visual acuity was reduced to 6/60 on the left, remaining normal on the right. There was also loss of colour vision on the left and a left relative afferent pupillary defect. Her symptoms improved within 4 weeks. Two years later, her left leg became numb. Within 1 week, the numbness had spread to involve the right leg and extended upwards to her waist, sparing the perineum. Examination at that time revealed a persistent left relative afferent pupillary defect, though visual acuity had returned to normal on that side, and a pale left optic disc on fundoscopy. There were no abnormal motor signs in the limbs, but she had impaired pinprick and temperature sensation in the legs with a level at T10.

Comment: This patient's clinical presentation is virtually pathognomonic of MS, even in the absence of results of laboratory investigations. Her initial left optic neuritis and subsequent cord involvement fulfil the clinical diagnostic criteria of two lesions in the central nervous system separated in time and space. There is a rare condition, known as Devic's disease (neuromyelitis optica), where patients suffer repeated episodes of optic neuropathy and cord lesions, the remainder of the CNS being relatively unaffected. However, this disease may be distinguished from MS in several ways, including the clinical pointer that the optic nerve and cord lesions are usually much more severe in Devic's disease, with less likelihood of recovery. Optic neuropathy in Devic's disease tends also to be bilateral. An auto-antibody has now been identified in the serum of most patients with Devic's disease.

Chapter 17

Nerve and muscle

Peripheral nerve disorders

Definitions

Mononeuropathy – peripheral nerves may be affected individually by trauma, particularly pressure, or by damage to their blood supply (the **vasa nervorum**).

Systemic disorders that generally render nerves excessively sensitive to pressure, e.g. diabetes mellitus, or that produce widespread compromise of their vasculature, e.g. vasculitic diseases, may lead to a **multifocal** neuropathy (or **mononeuritis multiplex**).

Polyneuropathy – multiple peripheral nerves are more commonly affected by inflammatory, metabolic or toxic processes that lead to a diffuse, distal, symmetrical pattern of damage usually affecting the lower limbs before the upper limbs.

Mononeuropathies

The common mononeuropathies are the following.

Carpal tunnel syndrome

Compression of the median nerve at the wrist, as it passes through the carpal tunnel, may occur:

Lecture Notes: Neurology, 9th edition. By Lionel Ginsberg. Published 2010 by Blackwell Publishing.

- in isolation, for example in patients with manual occupations,
- in disorders that render the nerve sensitive to pressure, e.g. diabetes mellitus,
- when the carpal tunnel is 'crowded' with excessive or abnormal soft tissue (Table 17.1).

The clinical features of carpal tunnel syndrome are:

- pain in the hand or arm, especially at night, or on exertion,
- wasting and weakness of the muscles of the thenar eminence (see Fig. 5.2),
- sensory loss in the hand, in the distribution of the median nerve (Fig. 17.1),
- tingling paraesthesiae in the distribution of the median nerve following percussion of the palm in the region of the carpal tunnel (**Tinel's sign**) or maximum passive flexion of the wrist for 60 seconds (**Phalen's test**),
- the condition is often bilateral.

The diagnosis may be confirmed electrodiagnostically (Chapter 8) or by ultrasound of the wrist. Investigations into the cause, if not obvious, should include blood glucose, ESR and thyroid function.

Treatment options, depending on severity, include:

- splinting the hand, especially at night, in a position of partial wrist extension,
- local injection of the carpal tunnel with corticosteroids,

Table 17.1 General medical associations of carpal tunnel syndrome.

Pregnancy
Diabetes mellitus
Local deformity, e.g. secondary to osteoarthritis, fracture
Rheumatoid arthritis
Myxoedema
Acromegaly
Amyloidosis

• surgical decompression of the median nerve at the wrist.

Ulnar neuropathy

The ulnar nerve is subject to damage from pressure at several sites along its course, but particularly at the elbow.

Clinical features include:
• pain and/or tingling paraesthesiae radiating from the elbow down the forearm to the ulnar border of the hand,
• wasting and weakness of the intrinsic muscles of the hand (sparing the thenar eminence – Chapter 5),
• sensory loss in the hand in the distribution of the ulnar nerve (Fig. 17.1),

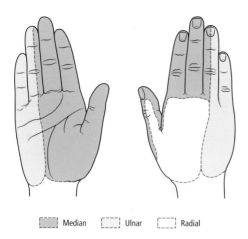

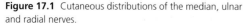

Figure 17.1 Cutaneous distributions of the median, ulnar and radial nerves.

• characteristic **claw hand deformity** in chronic lesions (Fig. 5.2).

Nerve conduction studies may localize the site of the lesion along the course of the ulnar nerve.

Mild lesions may respond to splinting of the arm at night, with the elbow extended to reduce pressure on the nerve. For more severe lesions, good results of surgical decompression, or ulnar nerve **transposition**, cannot be guaranteed. But operation is justified in the presence of continuing ulnar nerve damage, indicated by persisting pain and/or progressive motor impairment.

Radial palsy

Pressure on the radial nerve in the upper arm may lead to an acute **wrist drop** (Chapter 5) and sometimes sensory loss in the distribution of the superficial radial nerve (Fig. 17.1). Typically, the lesion is a consequence of a prolonged period of abnormal posture of the upper arm, e.g. draped awkwardly over an armchair because of alcohol intoxication ('**Saturday night palsy**').

Brachial plexus lesions

In addition to acute trauma to the brachial plexus, e.g. traction as a result of birth injury or road accidents, usually involving motorcyclists (upper roots of plexus – **Erb's paralysis**; lower roots – **Klumpke's paralysis**), several more chronic syndromes are recognized.

Cervical rib

A cervical rib or band of fibrous tissue may compress the brachial plexus at the thoracic outlet. In the past, this condition was overdiagnosed and overtreated by operative intervention. Surgical exploration of the brachial plexus nowadays is best reserved for patients with progressive wasting and weakness of the intrinsic hand muscles, appropriate sensory loss (usually along the ulnar border of the hand) and support from electrodiagnostic studies. Imaging of the brachial plexus even by MRI is not usually of value. Radiographs may reveal a cervical rib, but compression may result from a fibrous band invisible on plain X-ray.

Pancoast tumour

Bronchogenic carcinoma at the lung apex may invade the lower roots of the brachial plexus producing progressive pain in the ipsilateral arm, distal wasting and weakness, and sensory loss, particularly in the C7, C8 and T1 dermatomes. There may be an associated **Horner's syndrome** as a result of involvement of pre-ganglionic sympathetic fibres. A similar pattern may develop with other primary and secondary tumours.

Particular diagnostic difficulties may arise with breast carcinoma if there has been previous local radiotherapy – involvement of the brachial plexus may be due to invasion by tumour or **radiation plexopathy**.

Acute brachial neuritis (also known as neuralgic amyotrophy or idiopathic brachial plexopathy)

This condition is usually characterized by severe pain in the shoulder and arm at the onset. There is usually no obvious cause but it may follow immunization or operation. When the pain subsides (after days or weeks) patchy wasting and weakness of periscapular and more distal upper limb muscles is apparent. Some muscle groups are particularly prone to being affected, e.g. serratus anterior, leading to **winging** of the scapula (Fig. 17.2). The disorder is more often unilateral than bilateral and sensory involvement may be minimal. Electrodiagnostic studies are generally surprisingly unhelpful, though there may be evidence of denervation in affected muscles. CSF is normal. There is no specific treatment and spontaneous recovery of upper limb function may take 18 months to 2 years, but is not guaranteed.

Meralgia paraesthetica

Compression of the lateral cutaneous nerve of the thigh as it passes under the inguinal ligament produces a characteristic pattern of sensory loss (Fig. 17.3). The onset of this condition is particularly associated with a change (increase *or* decrease) in the patient's weight.

Lateral popliteal palsy

The common peroneal nerve is liable to damage from pressure as it winds round the fibular neck,

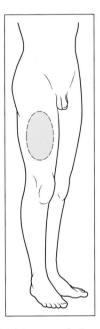

Figure 17.3 Meralgia paraesthetica. Distribution of sensory disturbance due to involvement of the lateral cutaneous nerve of the thigh.

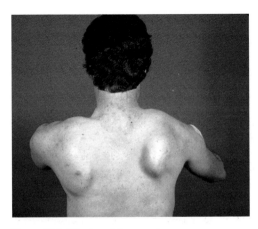

Figure 17.2 Winging of the scapula.

leading to a **foot drop**. There is weakness of ankle dorsiflexion and eversion, and of extensor hallucis longus, with variable sensory loss. The condition occurs commonly in immobile patients and in those whose nerves are prone to pressure, e.g. as a result of diabetes mellitus. A foot drop may also result from a lumbar root lesion (usually L5). Theoretically, this may be distinguished clinically from a peroneal nerve lesion as in the latter case inversion of the foot should be spared, tibialis posterior being supplied by the tibial not the peroneal nerve. However, electrodiagnostic studies are generally required to localize the lesion to the knee. Damage to the peroneal nerve is often reversible, being caused by conduction block (**neurapraxia**). Patients may meanwhile benefit from a **foot drop splint**.

Multifocal neuropathy

Causes of multifocal neuropathy (mononeuritis multiplex) include:
- malignant infiltration (carcinoma or lymphoma);
- vasculitis or connective tissue disease
  - rheumatoid arthritis,
  - systemic lupus erythematosus,
  - polyarteritis nodosa,
  - Wegener's granulomatosis;
- sarcoidosis;
- diabetes mellitus;
- infection
  - leprosy,
  - herpes zoster,
  - HIV,
  - Lyme disease;
- hereditary neuropathy with liability to pressure palsies.

Classically, multifocal neuropathy due to vasculitis presents with pain, weakness and sensory loss in the distribution of multiple peripheral nerves. The lower limbs are more commonly affected. Individual peripheral nerve lesions typically accumulate in a stepwise fashion acutely or subacutely, giving a clinical picture which is patchy and asymmetrical.

Polyneuropathy

Diffuse disease of the peripheral nerves may be subclassified according to whether there is sensory or motor involvement or both. Pathophysiologically, further subdivision is possible, depending on whether the site of disease is the myelin sheath or the nerve fibre itself (**demyelinating** and **axonal** neuropathies, respectively, distinguishable by nerve conduction studies). The causes of a polyneuropathy are summarized in Table 17.2.

Table 17.2 Causes of polyneuropathy.

Inherited
See Chapter 18
Infection
Leprosy
Diphtheria
Lyme disease
HIV
Inflammatory
Guillain–Barré syndrome (Chapter 20)
Chronic inflammatory demyelinating polyneuropathy
Sarcoid
Sjögren's syndrome
Vasculitis – lupus, polyarteritis
Neoplastic
Paraneoplastic (Chapter 19)
Paraproteinaemic
Metabolic
Diabetes mellitus
Uraemia
Myxoedema
Amyloid
Nutritional
Vitamin deficiency, especially thiamine, niacin and B_{12}
Toxic
For example, alcohol, lead, arsenic, gold, mercury, thallium, insecticides, hexane
Drugs
For example, isoniazid, vincristine, cisplatinum, metronidazole, nitrofurantoin, phenytoin, amiodarone

existent autonomic symptoms (Chapter 7). Clinical signs are those of widespread distal LMN involvement with muscle wasting, weakness and tendon areflexia. Distal position sense loss may result in **sensory ataxia**. There may be a characteristic **'glove-and-stocking'** distribution of impairment of pain, temperature and touch sensation (see Fig. 6.1b). Peripheral nerves may be thickened. Appropriate investigation of a patient presenting with a polyneuropathy is summarized in Table 17.3.

Treatment of polyneuropathy depends on the cause. Inflammatory neuropathies generally warrant management in specialist centres. Acute inflammatory demyelinating polyneuropathy

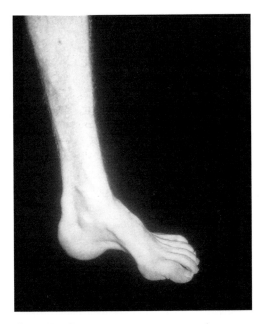

Figure 17.4 Pes cavus.

Patients may present with distal numbness and/or paraesthesiae or pain. Motor symptoms include distal weakness and wasting. Longstanding neuropathy may result in foot and hand deformity (**pes cavus**, Fig. 17.4; **claw hand**) and severe sensory loss may lead to **neuropathic ulceration** and joint deformity (Fig. 17.5). There may be co-

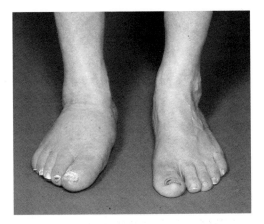

Figure 17.5 Neuropathic right ankle and foot (Charcot arthropathy).

Table 17.3 Investigation of polyneuropathy.

Blood tests
Full blood count, sedimentation rate, glucose, urea, electrolytes, liver and thyroid function, vitamin B_{12}, serum protein electrophoresis, auto-antibodies

Urine
Microscopy for evidence of vasculitis, glucose, porphyrins, Bence Jones protein

CSF
Raised protein, particularly in inflammatory neuropathies

Neurophysiology
Nerve conduction studies and EMG

Chest X-ray
For sarcoidosis, carcinoma

Special investigations for selected patients
Nerve biopsy, when the cause of a deteriorating neuropathy is unknown despite extensive investigation, also to confirm vasculitis, leprosy and chronic inflammatory demyelinating polyneuropathy
Bone marrow biopsy, skeletal survey for suspected myeloma

Specific blood tests for particular suspected conditions, e.g. DNA analysis for hereditary neuropathies, white cell enzymes for inborn errors of metabolism, *Borrelia* antibodies for Lyme disease

Table 17.4 Diseases causing demyelination, classified according to site and time course.

	Central nervous system	Peripheral nervous system
Acute	Acute disseminated encephalomyelitis (ADEM) (Chapter 16) – rare	Guillain–Barré syndrome (Chapter 20) – relatively common
Chronic	Multiple sclerosis (Chapter 16) – common	Chronic inflammatory demyelinating polyneuropathy (CIDP) – rare

(**Guillain–Barré syndrome**) is potentially a neurological emergency (Chapter 20). Chronic inflammatory demyelinating polyneuropathy (CIDP) and vasculitic neuropathies may require corticosteroid therapy and/or immunomodulatory measures, including immunosuppressant drugs (azathioprine, cyclophosphamide or cyclosporin), intravenous immunoglobulin or plasma exchange. Symptomatic treatment may alleviate neuropathic complications, including autonomic features (Chapter 7) and pain (Chapter 21).

It is important to distinguish Guillain–Barré syndrome and CIDP, both diseases of the peripheral nervous system, from demyelination in the CNS (Table 17.4).

Neuromuscular junction

Myasthenia gravis

This is an autoimmune disorder in which most patients have circulating antibodies to acetylcholine receptors at the neuromuscular junction

(Fig. 17.6). There may be associated thymus pathology (hyperplasia, atrophy or tumour – **thymoma**). The disease is rare, annual incidence is approximately 0.4 in 100,000, but with most patients surviving long term, prevalence is almost 1 in 10,000. All age groups may be affected.

Clinical features

These include:

- fatigable ptosis;
- diplopia with limitation of eye movements;
- facial weakness
  - **'myasthenic snarl'**,
  - weakness of eye closure;
- 'bulbar' symptoms and signs
  - dysphagia (with **nasal regurgitation** of liquids),
  - dysarthria (nasal quality);
- involvement of respiratory muscles (acute bulbar and respiratory symptoms caused by myasthenia gravis are a neurological emergency, Chapter 20);

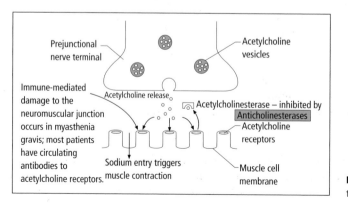

Prejunctional nerve terminal

Acetylcholine vesicles

Immune-mediated damage to the neuromuscular junction occurs in myasthenia gravis; most patients have circulating antibodies to acetylcholine receptors.

Acetylcholine release

Acetylcholinesterase – inhibited by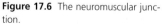

Acetylcholine receptors

Sodium entry triggers muscle contraction

Muscle cell membrane

Figure 17.6 The neuromuscular junction.

• neck and limb muscle weakness, worse at the end of the day and after exercise ('**fatigability**').

Investigations

• Serum acetylcholine receptor antibody analysis (15% of patients antibody negative – but, in some of these patients, other auto-antibodies may be identified).
• 'Tensilon' test: transient and rapid improvement in clinical features after intravenous injection of edrophonium (short-acting anticholinesterase temporarily preserves acetylcholine by blocking its metabolism). Test best performed 'double-blind', with atropine and cardiac resuscitation equipment available in view of muscarinic effects of excess acetylcholine.
• EMG, including single-fibre studies.
• Thyroid function tests for associated thyrotoxicosis.
• Striated muscle antibody analysis, positive in most patients with thymoma.
• CT scan of the anterior mediastinum, for thymic enlargement.

Treatment

• **Anticholinesterases**, e.g. pyridostigmine, provide symptomatic relief. However, patients requiring increasing doses may develop muscarinic cholinergic side effects, including increased salivation, vomiting, abdominal pain and diarrhoea. In extreme cases, weakness may worsen (**cholinergic crisis**, Chapter 20).
• **Corticosteroids**, e.g. prednisolone, are required for moderately severe disease unresponsive to other treatment. They are usually given as an alternate-day regime. Steroids should be gradually increased from a low dosage as symptoms may initially worsen. Hospital admission is generally advisable for starting steroids in patients whose disease is not purely ocular. Once control has been achieved, the dose may be tapered back in accordance with symptoms.
• **Immunosuppression**, e.g. with azathioprine, is used in combination with corticosteroids for moderately severe disease.

• **Thymectomy** for thymoma, and for younger patients early in the course of the disease to reduce requirements for medical therapy and, in a minority, achieve complete remission.
• **Plasma exchange** or intravenous immunoglobulin in preparation for thymectomy and in severe disease.

Certain antibiotics, such as aminoglycosides, should be avoided in myasthenic patients because of their blocking effect at the neuromuscular junction.

Other myasthenic syndromes

The neuromuscular junction may rarely be the site of congenital disease, or of a **paraneoplastic** disorder (**Lambert–Eaton myasthenic syndrome**, Chapter 19).

Myopathy

The causes of primary muscle disease are summarized in Table 17.5. In general, myopathies present clinically with weakness of the trunk and proximal limb muscles. There may also be dysphagia, weakness of neck flexion and/or extension, and of the muscles of facial expression. The gait is characteristically **waddling**. In acquired disorders, muscle wasting may be relatively mild at least in the early stages and the tendon reflexes spared. Investigation of primary muscle disease includes:
• blood tests
  • ESR, auto-antibodies (in acquired disease),
  • **creatine kinase** – released from damaged muscle cells;
• EMG – Chapter 8;
• muscle biopsy.

Specific disorders

Muscular dystrophies

Dystrophinopathies

Disease caused by mutations of the X-linked gene for the muscle protein **dystrophin** may present in childhood, or in adolescence or adult life.

Table 17.5 Causes of primary muscle disease.

Inherited
Muscular dystrophies
Metabolic myopathies

Infection
Gas gangrene
Staphylococcal myositis
Viral infection – especially influenza, Coxsackie,
 echo
Parasites – cysticercosis, trichinosis

Inflammation
Polymyositis
Dermatomyositis
Sarcoid

Neoplastic
Dermatomyositis – may be a paraneoplastic
 phenomenon (Chapter 19)

Metabolic (acquired)
Thyrotoxicosis
Cushing's syndrome
Osteomalacia

Toxic/drug induced
Corticosteroids
Halothane – 'malignant hyperpyrexia' (rare)
Other drugs may rarely be associated with
 myopathy

Degenerative
Inclusion body myositis

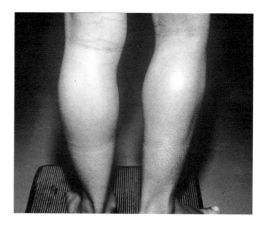

Figure 17.7 Calf pseudohypertrophy.

The childhood form (**Duchenne muscular dystrophy**) is severe. Affected boys typically develop proximal weakness in early childhood. They may have difficulty rising from a squatting position, using their hands to 'climb' up their legs (**Gowers' sign**). Calf muscles may show **pseudohypertrophy** (Fig. 17.7) because of replacement of muscle fibres with fatty connective tissue. Children are usually confined to a wheelchair before their teens. The disease progresses relentlessly, with death usually from cardiac and respiratory complications before the age of 20, though with better supportive care some patients are now surviving into early adult life. Less severe mutations may present in adolescence or adult life (**Becker muscular dystrophy**) and be compatible with

a normal lifespan, though often with progressive disability. Distinction from other **limb-girdle dystrophies** is now possible through molecular analysis of the dystrophin gene.

Other muscular dystrophies

Myotonic dystrophy is an autosomal dominant disorder in which patients characteristically have abnormally sustained muscle contraction or **myotonia**. This may manifest as inability to release the grip. Clinically, striking a muscle with a patellar hammer may elicit **percussion myotonia** and the condition may also be diagnosed by electromyography. There are other typical features:
• bilateral ptosis,
• facial weakness,
• wasting and weakness of sternomastoids,
• cataracts,
• endocrine associations, including diabetes mellitus, frontal balding and testicular atrophy.

Myotonia may be treated with phenytoin or mexiletine. It may also occur with relatively little muscle wasting or weakness in **myotonia congenita**.

Facioscapulohumeral muscular dystrophy is also usually an autosomal dominant condition. Patients have bilateral facial weakness and winging of both scapulae. In addition to weakness and wasting of proximal upper limb muscles there is typically weakness of the spinal and pelvic muscles, patients having a waddling gait and pronounced lumbar lordosis. Rarer muscular dystrophies and **congenital myopathies** may affect the extraocular and pharyngeal muscles.

Other inherited disorders

Metabolic defects, e.g. **glycogen storage diseases**, may produce muscle weakness, often with pain and cramps.

Mitochondrial myopathies are discussed in Chapter 18.

In **familial periodic paralysis**, bouts of profound muscle weakness, sometimes provoked by exercise, a high carbohydrate meal or exposure to cold, may be associated with hypo- or hyperkalaemia.

Acquired disorders

Inflammatory myopathies

Polymyositis may occur in isolation or in association with autoimmune connective tissue disorders, e.g. systemic sclerosis, fibrosing alveolitis and Sjögren's syndrome.

Dermatomyositis is the association of an inflammatory myopathy with a characteristic lilac (**heliotrope**) rash affecting the face. A purple-red rash may also involve the knuckles, anterior chest wall and other sites, particularly extensor surfaces. In a minority of patients with dermatomyositis, particularly males older than 45 years, there is an underlying malignancy, e.g. carcinoma of the bronchus or stomach.

Clinical features of inflammatory myopathies are those of a proximal myopathy, but there may be dysphagia as a result of pharyngeal muscle involvement, and muscle pain and tenderness. Arthralgia and Raynaud's phenomenon may occur.

Treatment, following histological confirmation, is with corticosteroids and immunosuppressant drugs, e.g. azathioprine, patients requiring monitoring for several years and most being left with some muscle weakness. One histological variant, **inclusion body myositis**, is particularly unresponsive to treatment. This condition, a relatively common cause of acquired muscle disease, typically affects older men. There is characteristic selective involvement of the finger flexors and quadriceps muscles. The lack of response to immunomodulatory therapy has led to the view that inflammatory changes are secondary to an underlying degenerative process in the muscles.

Key points

- Peripheral nerve disorders include mononeuropathies, multifocal neuropathies and polyneuropathies
- Myasthenia gravis is an autoimmune disorder of the neuromuscular junction characterized clinically by fatigable weakness typically affecting the extraocular and bulbar muscles
- Primary muscle disease (myopathy) usually presents with proximal weakness. Relevant investigations include serum creatine kinase, EMG and muscle biopsy. Disorders may be inherited (e.g., muscular dystrophies) or acquired (e.g., polymyositis)

Myasthenia gravis

Case history: A 48-year-old woman presented with a 6-week history of drooping eyelids, worse on the left and in the evenings, when she also experienced double vision. For 1 week before her admission to hospital, she had increasing difficulty chewing and swallowing her food, again worse in the evening, when she also developed slurred speech. There had been no choking but on one occasion she had experienced nasal regurgitation while drinking. She had previously been well and there was no family history of neurological disease, though there was a family history of thyroid disease. On examination, she had bilateral fatigable ptosis, more marked on the left and incomplete bilateral external ophthalmoplegia (i.e., involving the extraocular muscles, not the pupils). There was bilateral weakness of eye closure (orbicularis oculi) and, to a lesser extent, weakness of the other muscles of facial expression. She had a weak, transverse, smile. There was weakness of jaw opening and closure, and neck flexion and extension. She had fatigable dysarthria with a nasal quality, and palatal weakness. In the upper limbs, there was mild bilateral fatigable weakness, without wasting, of deltoid, triceps and finger extension. Lower limb power was normal. Tendon reflexes were symmetrically brisk with downgoing plantar responses. Sensory testing was normal, as was her gait.

Comment: This patient presents the typical pattern of severe generalized myasthenia, with fatigability and ocular, bulbar and limb involvement. The family history of organ-specific autoimmune disease is also noteworthy. The combination of an ophthalmoplegia with weakness of orbicularis oculi indicates myasthenia until proved otherwise. She requires urgent admission to hospital with close monitoring, including bedside tests of respiratory function (vital capacity). The pace of her history puts her at risk of a myasthenic crisis (Chapter 20). Other aspects of her initial management include a speech and language therapist's assessment of her swallowing and a course of intravenous immunoglobulin to 'buy time' while investigations are carried out and long-term management instituted (see main text).

See also Multifocal neuropathy in systemic vasculitis (Chapter 19) and Guillain–Barré syndrome (Chapter 20).

Chapter 18

Development and degeneration

Some neurological disorders are a consequence of a pathological insult to the nervous system during intrauterine development, at the time of birth or in the immediate postnatal period. Such conditions are, by definition, static in terms of the underlying pathology, though clinical features may become manifest only in childhood, adolescence or even later.

A second group of diseases arises from specific gene mutations, with a clear-cut pattern of inheritance – autosomal or sex-linked, dominant or recessive. These conditions may be recognizable at birth, but in many the onset is again delayed to childhood, adolescence or adult life. The underlying pathology tends to be progressive rather than static.

In a third group of conditions, overlapping with the second, there is progressive degeneration of specific parts of the nervous system, which may be partially genetically determined, but other factors contribute to the aetiology.

Lecture Notes: Neurology, 9th edition. By Lionel Ginsberg. Published 2010 by Blackwell Publishing.

Congenital disorders

Cerebral palsy

Definition and aetiology

A range of predominantly motor neurological deficits may arise from pre- or perinatal insults, sometimes in combination with learning difficulties, behavioural problems and epilepsy, but often compatible with survival into adult life. Risk factors for cerebral palsy are summarized in Table 18.1; of these prematurity is the most important.

Clinical features

Various patterns of disability are recognized:
- **Spastic diplegia** (Little's disease) – a congenital spastic paraparesis, sometimes with shortening and deformity of the legs contributing to the walking difficulty. The upper limbs are relatively spared, though there may be clumsiness of the hands.
- **Spastic hemiplegia** – a common form, often associated with hemianopic and hemisensory deficits, learning difficulties and epilepsy.
- **Athetoid cerebral palsy** – choreoathetoid movements developing in early childhood; children usually have normal cognitive function, though communication may be difficult because of dysarthria. In the past, a severe form of this

147

Table 18.1 Risk factors for cerebral palsy.

Antenatal
Fetal hypoxia or infection
Developmental abnormalities
Twins
Maternal (and paternal) age

Perinatal
Prematurity
Postmaturity
Traumatic delivery with neonatal intracranial
  haemorrhage

Postnatal
Preterm infants – hypoxia, hypoglycaemia, cerebral
  ischaemia or haemorrhage, hypothermia
Full-term infants – infection, trauma, kernicterus

syndrome was caused by neonatal hyperbilirubinaemia (**kernicterus**).
• **Other forms** may be more severe (tetraplegia), purely ataxic or mixed.

Management

The treatment of cerebral palsy includes surgical correction of associated squints and anti-epilepsy medication as required. Despite physiotherapy, contractures and other deformities may require orthopaedic intervention. Many children have special educational needs.

Spinal dysraphism

Definitions

Failure of normal closure of the **neural tube** during embryological development, along with a defect of the overlying skin and abnormal development of the bony structures, make up **dysraphism**. If the brain is involved, such lesions may be incompatible with life, as in **anencephaly**, where the brain and cranial vault are absent.

Spinal **dysraphism** varies in severity and particularly affects the lumbosacral region. In a spinal **myelomeningocoele**, parts of the spinal cord are extruded in a meningeal sac in the lumbosacral area, associated with paraplegia and

incontinence in severe cases. **Meningocoeles** contain meningeal tissue in the sac but no neural elements. Both these anomalies are associated with hydrocephalus (see below). **Spina bifida occulta** is the mildest form of dysraphism, where there is a failure of fusion of the vertebral arch(es) but no sac. A lumbar tuft of hair, dimple, pit or sinus may overlie the defect. In many normal individuals, failure of fusion of a vertebral arch is an incidental radiological finding.

Aetiology

The cause of neural tube defects is unknown, but several risk factors have been identified:
• history of neural tube defect in a sibling,
• trisomy 13 or 18,
• folate deficiency in early pregnancy,
• increase in risk associated with some anti-epilepsy drugs in pregnancy, particularly sodium valproate.

Management

Treatment of severe anomalies in neonates involves complex surgery and poses ethical problems, as surviving children are generally very severely disabled. The condition can now be diagnosed antenatally by fetal ultrasound examination, and elevated maternal serum and amniotic fluid alpha-fetoprotein levels.

Spina bifida occulta may present later in life with recurrent bacterial meningitis as a result of the presence of a sinus linking a skin dimple with the meninges. Alternatively, patients may develop a partial cauda equina syndrome. Investigation by MRI (Fig. 18.1) may reveal a tethered cord or an intraspinal lipoma or haemangioma in association with the bony defect, for which surgery can prevent further progression.

Infantile hydrocephalus

Aetiology

Congenital hydrocephalus is frequently associated with dysraphism and with other congenital malformations, including:
• cerebral aqueduct stenosis,

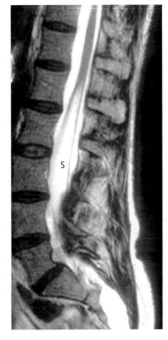

Figure 18.1 Spinal MRI showing tethered spinal cord, extending low into the lumbar theca. The elongated cord contains a fluid-filled cavity – a lumbar syrinx (s). Two parasagittal scans are shown, because of the patient's scoliosis.

- **Dandy–Walker syndrome** – outflow obstruction to the fourth ventricle with associated failure of development of the cerebellar vermis,
- **Arnold–Chiari malformation** – herniation of cerebellar tissue and sometimes the lower part of the brainstem through the foramen magnum.

Other factors may contribute to the development of hydrocephalus in the neonatal period, including trauma, haemorrhage, meningitis and, rarely, tumours.

Clinical features

Enlargement of the head may occur *in utero*, obstructing labour. More usually, infants appear normal at birth but subsequently show:
- progressive enlargement of the head (which can occur in infancy as the cranial sutures have not yet fused), with a tense anterior fontanelle, thin scalp with dilated veins and a 'cracked pot' skull percussion note,
- lid retraction and impaired upgaze, giving the eyes a 'setting sun' appearance,
- delayed development, learning difficulties, seizures, optic atrophy, spastic paraparesis.

Management

The diagnosis of hydrocephalus, if not clinically obvious, may be suspected from accurate successive head circumference measurements, and confirmed by skull radiograph or more usefully by CT cranial scan. Shunting the ventricles is usually required to prevent further deterioration. Other neurosurgical procedures will depend on the cause, e.g. foramen magnum decompression for Arnold–Chiari malformation. In some children with infantile hydrocephalus, the ventricular enlargement may spontaneously 'arrest', the patient surviving without treatment into adult life, though usually with severe physical and mental deficits.

Cerebral structural anomalies

Numerous malformations of the brain itself have been described; many may be incidental findings, e.g. **porencephalic cysts** communicating with the ventricles, whereas others may delay development and be associated with neurological deficits and epilepsy.

Intrauterine infection

With increased uptake of rubella immunization, and screening in pregnancy for rubella and syphilis, congenital infections are increasingly rare.

Congenital rubella is characterized by cataracts, hearing loss, severe learning difficulties and congenital heart disease.

Congenital neurosyphilis resembles the adult disease (Chapter 14) but with more rapid progression and certain specific features – deafness, interstitial keratitis and deformed teeth.

Neurogenetics

Most parts of the neuraxis are 'targets' for genetic defects, which may selectively damage specific cell populations, or may exert more diffuse effects. With advances in molecular genetics, the diagnosis of many of these conditions can now be confirmed by DNA analysis.

Cerebral cortex

Both Alzheimer's disease (AD) and prion disease may be inherited (see below).

Basal ganglia

Huntington's disease

This autosomal dominant disorder is characterized in its most typical form by progressive chorea and dementia, with an age of onset of 35–40 years. There is also a juvenile form where rigidity predominates over chorea (Westphal variant). Though the chorea may be partially alleviated by drugs, the condition is relentless, death ensuing usually within 15 years. Pathologically, there is atrophy of the caudate nucleus, along with more generalized cerebral atrophy. The disease mutation can now be detected directly by DNA analysis. This development has posed enormous ethical issues, because of the devastating implications of a positive diagnosis for the patient and their entire family. It is important to distinguish between **diagnostic testing**, to confirm the diagnosis in a patient suspected of having the condition, and **predictive testing** (testing a relative at risk). Individuals requesting the latter should be referred for specialist **genetic counselling**.

Wilson's disease

This is a rare autosomal recessive defect of copper metabolism. Levels of serum copper and cerulo-plasmin, the copper transport protein, are low and copper is deposited in the tissues, particularly the liver and basal ganglia. The disease may present in childhood with cirrhosis, or in adolescence, where the neurological features dominate. These include an akinetic–rigid syndrome, dystonia, cerebellar signs or sometimes neuropsychiatric manifestations, even frank psychosis. Copper is also deposited in the cornea, as **Kayser–Fleischer rings**, detectable on slit-lamp examination. The diagnosis of Wilson's disease, based on serum copper and caeruloplasmin, Kayser–Fleischer rings, increased urinary copper excretion and, if necessary, liver biopsy, is important, as the condition is treatable and is fatal without therapeutic intervention. The mainstay of treatment is penicillamine, a copper-chelating drug.

Cerebellum

Friedreich's ataxia

This rare autosomal recessive disorder presents in childhood with progressive ataxia, tendon areflexia and upgoing plantar responses. Skeletal deformities including kyphoscoliosis and pes cavus are generally found, as are electrocardiographic abnormalities, indicative of underlying cardiomyopathy, which is the usual cause of early death in this condition. DNA diagnosis is now available.

Late-onset ataxia

A number of conditions, generally with autosomal dominant inheritance and preserved tendon reflexes (hence distinct from Friedreich's ataxia), present in adult life with a progressive cerebellar syndrome. DNA testing is possible for several

Table 18.2 Differential diagnosis of cerebellar ataxia.

Inherited Friedreich's ataxia Other hereditary ataxias
Congenital Cerebellar hypoplasia Arnold–Chiari malformation Dandy–Walker syndrome
Trauma
Infection Cerebellar abscess Tuberculosis Postviral, e.g. varicella in childhood
Inflammation Multiple sclerosis
Neoplastic Cerebellar astrocytoma, haemangioblastoma,   metastases Paraneoplastic
Vascular Infarction Haemorrhage
Metabolic Myxoedema (rarely)
Toxic/drug induced Alcohol Phenytoin
Degenerative Multiple system atrophy

of these spinocerebellar ataxias. The differential diagnosis of cerebellar ataxia is given in Table 18.2.

Corticospinal tract

Hereditary spastic paraplegia

This is a disorder characterized by progressive spastic paraparesis, often apparent in childhood, with a typical 'scissoring' gait, and associated skeletal deformities, including pes cavus. In its 'pure' form, which is usually inherited with an autosomal dominant pattern, there is little or no clinical evidence of sensory involvement and sphincter

dysfunction occurs late, if at all. There are, however, various 'complicated' forms where the spastic paraparesis coexists with other deficits. Furthermore, autosomal recessive and sex-linked modes of inheritance are seen.

Optic nerve

Leber's hereditary optic neuropathy

This is a condition that typically presents in adolescence or early adult life with subacute unilateral then bilateral visual failure as a result of optic nerve disease. Patients are generally left with severe visual deficits. The disease is more common in males, for reasons that are unclear, as the underlying genetic defect is not sex-linked but is a mutation of mitochondrial DNA (see below).

Anterior horn cell

Hereditary spinal muscular atrophies

These specifically target anterior horn cells, with LMN signs of wasting and weakness in affected muscle groups. There are numerous variants, ranging from a fatal infantile form (**Werdnig–Hoffman disease**) to milder generalized disease presenting later in childhood or in adolescence (**Kugelberg–Welander disease**). Even milder forms may be confined to a single limb or show other focal distributions and a normal life expectancy. The pattern of inheritance is usually autosomal (or sex-linked) recessive.

Peripheral nerve

Charcot–Marie–Tooth disease (CMT)

CMT is the name given to a clinically and genetically heterogeneous group of disorders, rather than a single disease. These conditions are also known as hereditary motor and sensory neuropathy.

The most common variant in Western Europe (CMT1A) has an autosomal dominant pattern of inheritance, and can now be diagnosed by DNA analysis. Patients present with slowly progressive distal wasting and weakness, particularly affecting the anterolateral muscle compartment of the

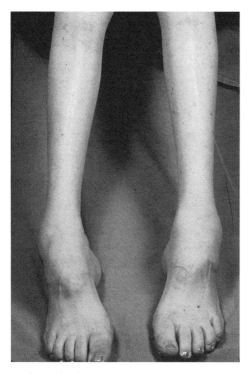

Figure 18.2 Charcot–Marie–Tooth disease.

Muscle

Muscular dystrophies

These may follow autosomal dominant, autosomal recessive or sex-linked patterns of inheritance. The major conditions are described in Chapter 17.

Other myopathies

Many other rare **congenital myopathies** have been reported, as have metabolic disorders that primarily affect muscle tissue. Of particular interest are the **mitochondrial** defects. These commonly arise from mutations of mitochondrial, as opposed to nuclear, DNA. Patients present with chronic progressive external ophthalmoplegia (superficially resembling ocular myasthenia) or combinations of multiple other neurological and systemic features, e.g. ataxia, dementia, neuropathy, epilepsy, retinitis pigmentosa, generalized myopathy, cardiomyopathy and lactic acidosis. Characteristic abnormalities may be seen with specialized staining of muscle biopsies ('**ragged red fibres**'). Mutations of mitochondrial DNA may be detectable in blood or muscle. Point mutations in the mitochondrial genome show a maternal pattern of inheritance, offspring receiving all their mitochondrial DNA from the ovum.

leg. This distribution, in combination with pes cavus, produces a characteristic appearance of the lower limbs (Fig. 18.2). Tendon reflexes are usually absent; sensory loss may be relatively mild. Peripheral nerves may be palpably thickened. Electrodiagnostic studies show marked slowing of nerve conduction velocities. Histological examination of peripheral nerve biopsies reveals segmental demyelination, in keeping with the electrical findings, and associated hypertrophy. CMT2 resembles type 1, but the age of onset may be later and nerve conduction velocity is relatively preserved, reflecting underlying axonal rather than demyelinating pathology. The prognosis of CMT is extremely variable, even within families. Some patients are wheelchair-bound by the time they reach middle age, whereas others are asymptomatic throughout a normal lifespan.

Other rarer genetic causes of a peripheral neuropathy may be associated with specific metabolic defects, e.g. familial amyloidosis, porphyria (Chapter 19) and the leucodystrophies (Chapter 16).

Neurogenetic tumour syndromes

Mutations in genes with presumed '**tumour suppressor**' function lead to disorders characterized by tumours, hamartomas, cysts and other abnormalities in multiple organs, but with a predilection for the nervous system. The major features of these conditions, which generally exhibit an autosomal dominant pattern of inheritance, are summarized in Table 18.3.

Neurodegeneration

One of the most common neurodegenerative disorders, Parkinson's disease, has been discussed in detail in Chapter 12. Others, with a clear-cut

Table 18.3 Neurogenetic tumour syndromes.

Disease	Nervous system	Skin	Other clinical features
Neurofibromatosis type 1 (von Recklinghausen disease)	Peripheral and spinal neurofibromas Optic nerve glioma Glioma Learning difficulties	Café-au-lait spots Dermatofibromas	Lisch nodules on iris Skeletal deformities Phaeochromocytoma
Neurofibromatosis type 2	Bilateral acoustic neuroma Meningioma Glioma Peripheral and spinal schwannomas	Few café-au-lait spots	Cataracts (usually asymptomatic)
Tuberous sclerosis	Learning difficulties Epilepsy Cerebral tubers and nodules Glioma	Adenoma sebaceum Subungual fibromas Hypopigmented patches Shagreen patches	Retinal phakomas Rhabdomyomas Renal cysts Renal angiolipomas
von Hippel–Lindau disease	Cerebellar haemangioblastoma (occasionally also spinal)		Retinal angiomas Renal cysts (also other organs) Renal carcinoma Phaeochromocytoma

Various other neurocutaneous syndromes should be considered separately from those listed in this table as they are neither associated with tumours, nor are they necessarily inherited. For example, Sturge–Weber syndrome consists of the combination of a cerebral arteriovenous malformation (with calcification) and a facial port-wine stain on the same side. Patients commonly present with epilepsy and contralateral hemiparesis.

genetic aetiology, are described above. The remainder of this chapter is concerned with two neuronal populations in the CNS that are subject to degenerative disease:

- cerebral cortex, in particular neurones involved in cognitive function,
- motor neurones (UMN and LMN).

Dementia

Dementia is defined as significant impairment (sufficient to interfere with normal work or social function) of two or more domains of cognition, one of which must be memory. There must be no evidence of delirium. Most patients with dementia have degenerative disease of the brain, though there are other causes (see below).

Alzheimer's disease

AD is the most common cause of dementia in all age groups, occurring with markedly increased frequency in the elderly. It is a neurodegenerative disorder characterized pathologically by intracellular **neurofibrillary tangles** composed of 'paired helical filaments', and extracellular **neuritic plaques** containing an amyloid core, along with neuronal loss (Fig. 18.3).

Aetiology and pathogenesis

Chemical analysis of the contents of neuritic plaques has revealed that their core is largely composed of a peptide, **amyloid beta-protein**, which is a fragment of a much larger protein, **amyloid precursor protein** (APP), encoded by a gene on chromosome 21. The central role of

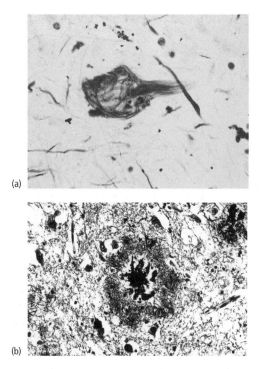

(a)

(b)

Figure 18.3 Alzheimer's disease – neuropathological hallmarks. (a) Neurofibrillary tangles, (b) neuritic plaques.

amyloid in AD pathogenesis has been established from rare instances of familial AD caused by a mutation in the APP gene. Observations on patients with Down's syndrome (trisomy 21) also support a pathogenetic role for amyloid, as these individuals develop premature features of AD and may be at risk of excess amyloid formation from their extra copy of the APP gene. But the cause(s) of AD must be more complex than amyloid formation alone, as the great majority of cases are non-familial, and in some familial examples, mutations have been identified in genes other than that coding for APP. A specific isoform of the lipid transport protein **apolipoprotein E** has been identified as an independent risk factor for the development of both familial and sporadic AD.

Regardless of the underlying molecular mechanisms, the end result of the pathogenetic process in AD is the death of neurones in specific areas

of the cerebral cortex concerned with aspects of cognition, notably the hippocampus and adjacent structures, and the temporal neocortex. Some deeper structures are also involved, e.g. the nucleus basalis of Meynert in the frontal lobe. Cholinergic neurones are particularly affected, providing a rationale for the use of cholinergic-enhancing drugs to improve memory in this disease.

Clinical features

Early in the course of the illness, memory loss is apparent, particularly for recent events. Patients have difficulty learning and retaining new information. The history is frequently obtained from near relatives rather than patients themselves, who may be unaware of their problems.

Later, the impairment of memory, along with attention deficits, leads to disorientation in time. There are word-finding difficulties and loss of general knowledge. Perceptual deficits may be accompanied by hallucinations and delusions. Finally, there is severe global loss of cognitive function – amnesia, dysphasia, dyspraxia and agnosia. Personality disintegrates with behavioural disturbances, incontinence, increasing dependence and death within 5–10 years.

Diagnosis

There is no specific test for AD in life. However, careful application of clinical diagnostic criteria is accurate in more than 80% of cases. It is important to exclude other causes of dementia, particularly those that might be amenable to treatment (Table 18.4).

Management

Systemic illness, e.g. infection, can exacerbate dementia; hence, attention should be paid to the patient's general health, including avoidance of sedative drugs (unless clearly indicated), alcohol and fatigue.

Simple memory aids are helpful early in the disease, e.g. labels, diaries. Patients should wear

Table 18.4 Causes of dementia.

Inherited
Familial Alzheimer's disease
Huntington's disease
Some cerebellar ataxias
Wilson's disease

Trauma
Subdural haematoma
Other severe head injuries

Infection
Syphilis
Subacute sclerosing panencephalitis
AIDS-related dementia
Progressive multifocal leucoencephalopathy
Cerebral Whipple's disease (associated with arthritis
  and gut symptoms)

Inflammation
Multiple sclerosis
Sarcoid, lupus, vasculitis

Neoplasm
Frontal tumours
Multiple cerebral metastases
Hydrocephalus secondary to posterior fossa tumour
  (**NB:** normal-pressure hydrocephalus, in the absence
  of a structural cause, may present with dementia –
  see text)
Paraneoplastic

Vascular
Multi-infarct dementia

Metabolic
Myxoedema
Vitamin B$_{12}$ deficiency
Chronic organ failure – Chapter 19

Drugs/toxins
For example, barbiturates, alcohol, lead

Degenerative
Alzheimer's disease
Dementia with Lewy bodies
Frontotemporal dementia
Prion diseases – may also be considered both
  inherited and transmissible
Parkinson's disease and other akinetic–rigid syndromes
  (see text)

MedicAlert bracelets. The driver licensing authority should be notified.

Various cholinergic-enhancing drugs have been used to improve memory early in the disease, albeit for only a few months, most notably the cholinesterase inhibitors donepezil, rivastigmine and galantamine (the last is also an agonist at nicotinic receptors). Memantine affects glutamate transmission and is licensed for use in moderate to severe AD in the UK. No drugs are yet known to affect disease progression in AD. Furthermore, symptomatic treatment, e.g. with donepezil, should be continued only if the patient or more likely their carer(s) is aware of clear benefit to quality of life. Other drugs with a role in treating non-cognitive features in AD include antidepressants, neuroleptics and anxiolytics.

Later in the illness, with increasing dependence, the brunt of the patient's management often falls on the spouse or other near relative, usually themselves elderly, who act as carers with little respite. There are, however, external support services, e.g. psychiatric care in the community, day hospitals, opportunities for respite care and information from specialist organizations, e.g. the Alzheimer's Disease Society in the UK.

Other causes of dementia

Degenerative diseases

Prion diseases are a group of rare neurodegenerative disorders in animals and man, previously classified together largely on the basis of shared histological characteristics ('**spongiform encephalopathies**'). The archetypal human disorder, **Creutzfeldt–Jakob disease** (CJD), illustrates the remarkable characteristics common to these conditions in that it is potentially both inherited and transmissible.

The molecular basis for these phenomena resides in the infectious pathogen of the spongiform encephalopathies, termed the '**prion**'. This entity is unique in being composed entirely of protein (the **prion protein** [PrP]), with no evidence for a nucleic acid component, and is highly resistant to heat and formaldehyde. Furthermore, there is a normal isoform of PrP, present in uninfected cells, and encoded by a normal human gene. The precise chemical nature of the difference between the cellular and pathogenic isoforms of PrP remains unclear.

Most instances of CJD are sporadic, where the underlying mechanism may be somatic mutation of the PrP gene. Familial CJD (10–15% of cases) is inherited as an autosomal dominant trait, and is due to a point mutation of the PrP gene. Infectious CJD has been documented in various iatrogenic circumstances, e.g. following accidental inoculation of patients with prions at surgery, or from corneal grafts, or the use of growth hormone made from human pituitary extract. These instances show the incubation period for CJD to be very long – usually several years. Intense research and media interest and concern in these conditions, despite their rarity, has been stimulated by a variant of CJD, attributed to human consumption of prion-contaminated beef (bovine spongiform encephalopathy).

Clinically, CJD is characterized by a rapidly progressive dementia, death usually ensuing within 1–2 years or less, sometimes associated with cortical visual problems and motor features, e.g. myoclonus, and occasionally muscle wasting and fasciculation. Variant CJD occurs in younger patients and initially presents with psychiatric features, sensory disturbance and ataxia before the onset of dementia. The EEG in classical CJD may show a characteristic abnormality, '**periodic complexes**'. Neuroimaging is relatively normal in these conditions, though a characteristic appearance of the thalamus on MR has been described in many patients with variant CJD. The CSF may contain elevated levels of neuronal proteins, but the diagnosis can only be confirmed by biopsy (brain or lymphoid tissue – tonsil) or at autopsy. There is no proven treatment for the spongiform encephalopathies.

Other degenerative dementias may be distinguished from AD by different histological appearances of the brain at autopsy. Furthermore, the neurodegeneration in some of these conditions tends to be confined, at least initially, to the frontal or temporal lobes (frontotemporal dementias). Patients therefore present with **dementia of frontal type** – changes in personality, social behaviour and higher executive function (Chapter 3), often associated with a progressive non-fluent dysphasia (as a result of focal frontal lobe atrophy). Alternatively, they may develop **semantic dementia**, with word-finding difficulties and loss of general knowledge (as a result of focal temporal lobe atrophy). The progressive dysphasia in these latter patients remains fluent. Frontotemporal dementia is more likely to be encountered in younger patients.

Dementia may also be associated with movement disorders, e.g. Huntington's disease and progressive supranuclear palsy (Chapter 12). In these instances, the dementia is often described as '**subcortical**', with prominent slowing of cognitive function (**bradyphrenia**), personality and mood changes, and relative absence, at least initially, of the focal cortical deficits (e.g., dysphasia, dyspraxia and agnosia) so typical of AD.

Some degenerative dementias show a mixture of cortical and subcortical features. In particular, **dementia with Lewy bodies** (DLB) is recognized as a relatively common neurodegenerative cause of dementia, second only to AD. Lewy bodies are the major histological features of Parkinson's disease when confined to nigrostriate neurones (Chapter 12), but in this condition, as the name implies, they are more widely distributed. Distinguishing features of DLB include:

- fluctuating cognition with nocturnal confusion,
- visual hallucinations,
- evidence of Parkinsonism,
- worsening of clinical features with neuroleptic and antiparkinsonian drugs, even in small doses.

Patients with apparently straightforward idiopathic Parkinson's disease not uncommonly develop dementia some years after the onset of the movement disorder (Parkinson's disease with dementia [PDD]). In such circumstances, it can be difficult to know whether the patient has AD superimposed on Parkinson's disease or has developed more widespread Lewy body changes. Arbitrarily, patients are said to have DLB if the movement disorder and dementia present within a year of each other, and PDD if the onset of dementia is delayed by more than a year after the emergence of Parkinsonism.

Non-degenerative causes of dementia

Vascular (multi-infarct) dementia

This is a relatively common condition, caused by recurrent thromboembolism from extracranial sources or, more commonly, small vessel disease in the brain (Chapter 11). Clinical features suggesting vascular dementia include:
- abrupt onset and stepwise progression, unlike the typical gradual progression of AD,
- presence of vascular disease elsewhere and of vascular risk factors,
- combined cortical and subcortical deficits,
- nocturnal confusion, fluctuating cognition,
- emotional lability and other features of pseudo-bulbar palsy (Chapter 4).

Treatment of multi-infarct dementia is limited to management of vascular risk factors, in an attempt to avoid further progression.

Other non-degenerative causes of dementia are listed in Table 18.4. Many of these are potentially amenable to treatment. Two conditions, for which surgical treatments are available, warrant more detailed consideration.

Chronic subdural haematoma

This occurs predominantly in the elderly and may follow relatively minor head injury. Indeed, a history of trauma is not always obtainable, perhaps in part because of the delay (months or even years) before presentation. The typical clinical setting is in an elderly patient, predisposed to haematoma formation by cerebral atrophy and hence stretching of veins in the subdural space. Minor head trauma, e.g. in the context of alcoholism, may trigger bleeding, especially in a patient who is prone to recurrent haemorrhage because of a coagulation defect.

Pathologically, a gradually expanding cavity develops, filled with yellow or brown fluid as a result of breakdown of blood, and surrounded by a membrane. The mechanism of enlargement of

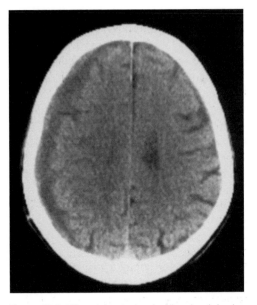

Figure 18.4 CT cranial scan showing chronic subdural haematoma.

the haematoma with time was originally thought to involve protein degradation and hence increasing osmotic pressure within the cavity, but recurrent bleeding is now judged the more important pathogenetic factor. The expanding haematoma exerts mass effect with shift of midline structures (unless bilateral subdural haematomas are present).

Clinically, patients may present solely with dementia but there may also be fluctuations in conscious level, epilepsy, signs of raised intracranial pressure and focal neurological deficits.

The diagnosis is usually apparent on CT cranial scan (Fig. 18.4), though difficulties may arise early in the course of the condition, when the haematoma is isodense with brain tissue, particularly if bilateral lesions are present and hence there is no midline shift. Treatment is by surgical evacuation of the haematoma through burr holes, often with dramatic benefit.

Normal-pressure hydrocephalus

This is suggested by the classic clinical triad of:
- dementia,

- gait disturbance,
- early urinary incontinence.

Gross ventricular enlargement without cortical atrophy is seen on CT cranial scanning and lumbar puncture reveals normal CSF pressure. The pathogenesis of the condition is obscure. Though a single reading of CSF pressure at lumbar puncture is likely to be normal, continuous intracranial pressure monitoring over 1–2 days may reveal waves of raised pressure. Results of surgical treatment by ventriculoperitoneal shunting are variable.

Motor neurone disease

Motor neurone disease (alternatively known as **amyotrophic lateral sclerosis**) is a progressive degenerative disorder of cortical, brainstem and spinal motor neurones (i.e., both UMNs and LMNs).

Epidemiology

The incidence of motor neurone disease is 2 per 100,000 per year. There is a slight male preponderance (1.5:1) and the condition is more common in the middle-aged and elderly, with peak onset at around 60 years. Approximately 5–10% of patients have a family history, suggestive of autosomal dominant inheritance, with a younger age of onset in these individuals. Among the familial patients, a proportion have identified mutations in the gene for the enzyme superoxide dismutase.

Aetiology and pathogenesis

Two mechanisms of motor neurone degeneration are currently considered likely to contribute to the pathogenesis of this disease:
- **excitotoxicity** – toxins interacting with glutamate receptors, resulting in cellular calcium overload;
- **free radicals** – motor neurone damage by a cascade of reactions initiated by electron capture by oxygen free radicals, e.g. superoxide and peroxide.

These two mechanisms may act together. Thus, oxygen free radicals are generated in response to a rise in intracellular calcium, which may in turn be induced by unidentified excitotoxins.

Clinical features and prognosis

Patients typically present with wasting and weakness of upper limb, more commonly than lower limb, muscles. Cramps and fasciculation may precede other motor symptoms. Examination shows a combination of LMN and UMN signs. The diagnosis is straightforward when such signs coexist in the same region (e.g., wasted arms with brisk upper limb reflexes) and several regions (cranial nerves, arms, legs) are affected, with evidence of disease progression. However, difficulties may arise early in the evolution of the illness, when only LMN or UMN signs are present in one limb. Furthermore, 10% of patients show only LMN signs throughout (formerly termed the 'progressive muscular atrophy' variant).

Motor signs are usually asymmetrical, at least initially. Sensory signs are absent, and there is no sphincter involvement beyond constipation caused by pelvic and abdominal muscle weakness and reduced fluid intake. A few patients develop dementia of frontal type.

A minority of patients present with dysarthria and dysphagia (the 'progressive bulbar palsy' variant). Signs of a mixed bulbar and pseudobulbar palsy are present, e.g. a wasted, fasciculating tongue but brisk jaw reflex. These patients are at risk of chest infection as a result of aspiration, compounded by ventilatory muscle weakness. These complications also develop in patients presenting with limb involvement, as the majority progress to bulbar symptoms. Other features of advanced disease include:
- depression, with increasing social isolation,
- weight loss, malnutrition and dehydration because of dysphagia,
- venous thromboembolism, because of immobility,
- ventilatory failure, the usual cause of death.

The median survival in motor neurone disease is 4 years, with a worse prognosis in patients with bulbar onset. Only 10% of patients survive 5 years or more, those with only LMN signs having a better outlook.

Investigations and diagnosis

Blood tests are usually normal apart from possible modest elevation of creatine kinase.

EMG typically reveals widespread evidence of denervation as a result of anterior horn cell damage. Nerve conduction studies exclude a motor neuropathy masquerading as motor neurone disease with purely LMN features.

Spinal imaging by MR may be needed to exclude cord or root compression.

Bulbar disease with solely LMN features may mimic myasthenia gravis, which may require formal exclusion by appropriate investigation (Chapter 17), as it is eminently treatable. Unlike myasthenia, motor neurone disease only very rarely involves eye movements.

Because of the grave prognostic implications, motor neurone disease should be diagnosed with certainty only on the basis of strict clinical criteria, ideally coexistent LMN and UMN signs in several regions, with evidence of progression. All other cases are only possible, or at worst probable, motor neurone disease, and care should be taken to exclude other potentially treatable conditions.

Management

Drug treatment

Most drug treatment is symptomatic:
- anticholinergic drugs for reducing saliva secretion when swallowing is difficult (other approaches to this problem include injection of botulinum toxin into the salivary glands),
- baclofen, dantrolene, tizanidine, diazepam for spasticity,
- quinine for cramp,
- antidepressants,
- laxatives (with increased fluids) for constipation,
- opiates, diazepam – terminally for symptomatic relief of dyspnoea.

The excitotoxicity theory of motor neurone disease pathogenesis has yielded a drug, **riluzole**, with antiglutamate activity. This has been shown to prolong life in motor neurone disease, but only for a few months in selected patients.

Other measures

- Physiotherapy.
- Communication aids for dysarthria.
- Adaptations at home – assessed by an experienced occupational therapist.
- Advice from speech therapists and dietitians for dysphagia.
- More severe dysphagia may require gastrostomy to bypass the defective swallowing mechanism and permit adequate fluid and nutritional intake.
- Assisted ventilation for respiratory failure may be justified, e.g. for nocturnal support, when other aspects of motor function are relatively preserved, but raises ethical issues in patients with advanced disease where life may be prolonged but so may suffering.
- Hospice care may be required terminally.
- Information and patient support is provided by the Motor Neurone Disease Association in the UK.

Key points

- Congenital neurological disorders, e.g. cerebral palsy, generally have static rather than progressive underlying pathology, though they may present in adult life
- Neurogenetic diseases may selectively 'target' specific neuronal populations
- Neurodegenerative disorders, which may or may not be inherited, also typically result in selective neuronal damage
- Treatable causes of dementia should be excluded before arriving at a diagnosis of a neurodegenerative condition

---

Alzheimer's disease

Case history: A 70-year-old woman came to the clinic at her family's request. They were concerned about her memory, but she said she felt well and that her memory was no worse than that of her contemporaries. Her son remarked that the patient's cognitive problems began 2 years previously when she was widowed. At first, they were attributed to depression consequent on the bereavement and she was treated with antidepressants. Her mood improved but she remained forgetful and had difficulty with daily tasks, particularly handling money. Later she stopped attending all the social activities with which she had been involved. Her family noticed she was less careful about her personal appearance and housework, about both of which she had previously been meticulous. General examination was normal. Bedside tests of cognitive function showed her to be disorientated for the date and month but she knew the year and the day of the week. She was able to repeat three words given to her by the examiner but could not remember any of them 5 minutes later. She knew the name of the prime minister but not the leader of the opposition, and was unable to recall any recent news events. Though she could name a watch and a pen, she could not name the winder or nib. She could draw a clock face but could not place the hands on it. Neurological examination of her cranial nerves and limbs was normal. A diagnosis of probable AD was made. Routine blood tests were non-contributory, including thyroid function, syphilis serology and vitamin B_{12} estimation. CT cranial scan showed moderate cerebral atrophy but no focal lesion. She was started on donepezil. Six months later, her condition was stable. However, by 2 years after her presentation she was unable to manage independently, even with family support, and was moved to a nursing home where she could be supervised 24 hours a day.

Comment: There are several typical features of AD in this patient's case, including her age, the insidious onset, early involvement of memory and language function and negative results of general neurological examination and screening investigations. The patient's lack of awareness of problems which had concerned her family is characteristic of an 'organic' dementia. Though drugs such as donepezil can alleviate symptoms of AD temporarily, they do not influence the progression of the underlying disease process.

Motor neurone disease

Case history: A 65-year old man presented with a 3-month progressive history of speech and swallowing difficulties. His symptoms were worse in the evening, when his speech became slurred and he struggled to finish his meal. Abnormal examination findings at this stage consisted solely of fatigable dysarthria with a nasal quality to his speech. A presumptive clinical diagnosis of myasthenia gravis was made. Single-fibre EMG studies provided some support for this diagnosis, but he had no acetylcholine receptor antibodies in his blood. An edrophonium (Tensilon) test was not carried out due to cardiac risk. He was treated with pyridostigmine, an anticholinesterase, and oral corticosteroids in gradually increasing doses. There was no objective benefit. Three months later, his wife remarked that he had become more emotional than usual, easily being triggered into uncontrollable laughter or tears. Re-examination at this time revealed widespread fasciculation in all four limbs, even after pyridostigmine had been discontinued. His tongue was also fasciculating and moved slowly. The jaw reflex had become brisk, as were all the limb tendon reflexes, and both plantar responses were upgoing.

Comment: The main differential diagnosis of a pure bulbar (LMN) palsy lies between myasthenia gravis and motor neurone disease. This patient presented with fatigable dysarthria and dysphagia suggesting myasthenia, but the absence of acetylcholine receptor antibodies and lack of response to treatment were of concern. Single-fibre EMG studies provide helpful supportive evidence for a diagnosis of myasthenia but the findings need not be specific. Within 3 months he had developed pseudobulbar (UMN) features – emotional lability, slow tongue movements, brisk jaw reflex – and a mixture of LMN and UMN signs in the limbs. The diagnosis, therefore, had to be revised to motor neurone disease. Fasciculations are a recognised side effect of anticholinesterases.

Chapter 19

Neurology and other medical specialties

The interface between neurology and other branches of medicine often poses the greatest challenges in patient management, both diagnostically and therapeutically.

Metabolic encephalopathy

The metabolic causes of an acquired **acute encephalopathy**, presenting with confusion or coma, and sometimes seizures, are summarized in Table 19.1.

Chronic organ failure and other progressive systemic disorders may produce structural changes in the nervous system with a rather different, slowly evolving, clinical presentation, particularly affecting:
- cerebral cortex – amnesia and other cognitive deficits, which may fluctuate; behavioural abnormalities,
- basal ganglia – dyskinesias or an akinetic–rigid syndrome,
- cerebellum – dysarthria, ataxia.

There may be coexistent myelopathy, peripheral neuropathy and myopathy.

Though metabolic encephalopathies share many clinical manifestations, particular disorders are associated with some distinctive motor features. Thus, for example, tremor is typically

Lecture Notes: Neurology, 9th edition. By Lionel Ginsberg. Published 2010 by Blackwell Publishing.

a component of alcohol withdrawal (see below). Myoclonic jerking is seen in renal failure and respiratory alkalosis. **Asterixis**, in many ways the opposite of myoclonus, is characterized by abrupt, transient, repeated wrist and finger flexion ('flapping tremor') caused by brief interruptions of muscle tone. Classically, it occurs in hepatic encephalopathy, but it is also seen in renal and respiratory failure.

Other metabolic processes warrant more detailed description.

Vitamin deficiencies

The neurological consequences of individual vitamin deficiencies are summarized in Table 19.2. Of these, vitamin B_1 (thiamine) deficiency produces an important syndrome, in terms of both its clinical characteristics, and the need for urgent therapy.

Wernicke–Korsakoff syndrome

Acute thiamine deficiency is encountered in two classical contexts in developed countries:
- chronic alcoholism – with associated malnutrition,
- **hyperemesis gravidarum** – severe vomiting in early pregnancy, again resulting in malnutrition.

In both cases, the full-blown Wernicke–Korsakoff syndrome may be precipitated by the

Table 19.1 Metabolic causes of acute encephalopathy.

Hypoxia, e.g. due to cardiac arrest, profound hypotension
Hypoglycaemia
Organ failure – respiratory, renal or hepatic
Ionic disturbances – hypo- and hypernatraemia, disturbances of calcium or magnesium metabolism (more often produce a chronic encephalopathy)
Vitamin deficiency (Table 19.2)
Endocrine disorders (Table 19.4)
Toxins, e.g. carbon monoxide, lead, alcohol (see text)

Table 19.2 Neurological effects of vitamin deficiency.

Vitamin	Neurological deficit
B_1 (thiamine)	See text
B_3 (niacin)	Acute and chronic encephalopathy
	Cerebellar syndrome
	Myelopathy
B_6 (pyridoxine)	Polyneuropathy (as seen with isoniazid treatment if pyridoxine is not given simultaneously)
B_{12} (cobalamine)	Dementia
	Optic atrophy
	Polyneuropathy
	Subacute combined degeneration of the cord (damage to corticospinal tracts and posterior columns)
D (calciferol)	Myopathy
E (tocopherol)	Spinocerebellar degeneration

patient's admission to hospital and intravenous dextrose administration without concomitant thiamine replacement (thiamine is a coenzyme required for normal carbohydrate metabolism).

Clinically, **Wernicke's encephalopathy** is defined by the triad of:
- ophthalmoplegia – typically nystagmus, third and sixth nerve palsies,
- ataxia,
- confusion, ultimately coma.

There may be hypothermia, because of hypothalamic involvement. Vitamin B_1 deficiency also commonly leads to a peripheral neuropathy.

Korsakoff's psychosis may become apparent only when the acute features of Wernicke's encephalopathy have been treated. It is a relatively selective cognitive dysfunction, characterized by amnesia, particularly for recent events, with a tendency to **confabulation**, the patient supplying fictitious information to cover memory gaps.

Pathologically, in fatal cases of the Wernicke–Korsakoff syndrome, microhaemorrhages are visible in the brainstem and diencephalon. Retinal haemorrhages are sometimes seen on fundoscopy. Biochemical abnormalities include elevated blood pyruvate levels and reduced **erythrocyte transketolase** activity.

The diagnosis is primarily clinical, though these biochemical features may provide retrospective laboratory support. Thiamine treatment should be instituted urgently in suspected cases and given prophylactically in alcoholics presenting with an acute withdrawal syndrome, and in patients with hyperemesis gravidarum. Delayed therapy increases the likelihood of death or permanent neurological deficit. In particular, features of Korsakoff's psychosis are less likely to respond to thiamine replacement.

Alcohol and the nervous system

Apart from the Wernicke–Korsakoff syndrome, alcohol exerts many direct and indirect effects on the nervous system.

- Acute intoxication – the well-known features of drunkenness may progress with very high blood alcohol levels through amnesia, ataxia and dysarthria with sympathetic overactivity (tachycardia, mydriasis, flushing), ultimately to disorientation and, rarely, coma. At this stage, the patient is at risk of death more from vomiting and aspiration than from the direct toxic action of alcohol.
- Alcohol withdrawal – chronic alcoholics experience a syndrome following alcohol withdrawal characterized by restlessness, irritability, tremor,

frightening visual hallucinations, confusion and seizures (**delirium tremens**). Treatment is by sedation, along with fluid and electrolyte correction, adequate nutrition and thiamine prophylaxis against the Wernicke–Korsakoff syndrome.

Alcohol withdrawal seizures may also occur in non-alcoholics after a single bout of binge drinking.

- Chronic alcoholism is associated with progressive structural damage to the nervous system including:
  - cerebral atrophy – the resultant dementia may be exacerbated by coexistent depression, along with the effects of multiple seizures and head injuries (possibly complicated by subdural haematoma),
  - cerebellar degeneration – particularly characterized by gait ataxia,
  - optic atrophy (**alcoholic amblyopia**),
  - peripheral neuropathy – painful, predominantly sensory, sometimes with autonomic features,
  - myopathy.
- Liver damage in alcoholism may indirectly affect the brain in several ways:
  - acute encephalopathy in fulminant hepatic failure,
  - reversible hepatic encephalopathy (Table 19.3),

Table 19.3 Hepatic encephalopathy.

Symptoms
Reversal of normal sleep–wake cycle
Cognitive impairment – may fluctuate
Personality change
Slurred speech
Tremor

Signs
'Flapping' tremor (asterixis)
Constructional apraxia (Chapter 3)
Hypertonus, brisk tendon reflexes
Ultimately coma, with hyperventilation

Investigations
Psychometric assessment – in early stages
EEG – characteristic triphasic waves, slowing
Elevated blood ammonia concentration

- **hepatocerebral degeneration syndrome** – dementia, pyramidal and extrapyramidal signs with asterixis as a result of chronic portosystemic shunting of blood.

Chronic liver disease (not necessarily caused by alcohol) and associated hyponatraemia (particularly if corrected over-rapidly) may lead to **central pontine myelinolysis** (Chapter 16).

Porphyria

Acute intermittent porphyria is a rare inherited disorder of porphyrin metabolism in which patients experience episodes of neuropsychiatric disturbance associated with gastrointestinal symptoms. Attacks may be triggered by alcohol, oral contraceptives and drugs, particularly barbiturates and sulphonamides. An acute psychosis or encephalopathy coincides with a predominantly motor peripheral neuropathy and abdominal pain. The diagnosis is confirmed by testing the patient's urine for excess porphobilinogen. Treatment includes avoidance of triggers and management of an acute attack with high carbohydrate intake, and sometimes intravenous haematin, which both inhibit porphyrin synthesis, plus symptomatic measures such as phenothiazines for psychosis and benzodiazepines for seizures.

Endocrine disease

The neurological consequences of the major endocrine disorders are summarized in Table 19.4. Thyrotoxicosis and diabetes mellitus warrant more detailed discussion because of the range of complications.

Thyrotoxicosis

Thyrotoxicosis may affect many sites in the nervous system:
- Cerebral cortex
  - anxiety, psychosis, even encephalopathy in patients with hyper-acute severe disease ('thyroid storm'),
  - strokes, secondary to atrial fibrillation;

Disorder	Neurological syndrome
Acromegaly	Chronic encephalopathy Visual field defects (chiasmal compression by tumour) Carpal tunnel syndrome Obstructive sleep apnoea Myopathy
Hypopituitarism	Acute or chronic encephalopathy
Thyrotoxicosis	See text
Myxoedema	Acute or chronic encephalopathy Cerebellar syndrome Hypothermia Neuropathy, myopathy
Cushing's syndrome	Psychosis, depression Myopathy
Addison's disease	Acute encephalopathy
Hyper- and hypoparathyroidism	Encephalopathy, seizures Myopathy 'Benign intracranial hypertension' Tetany – with hypocalcaemia
Diabetes mellitus	See text
Insulinoma	Acute or chronic encephalopathy
Phaeochromocytoma	Paroxysmal headache (with hypertension) Intracranial haemorrhage (rarely)

Table 19.4 Neurological consequences of endocrine disease.

- Basal ganglia
  - chorea;
- Exaggerated physiological tremor;
- UMN
  - hyper-reflexia;
- Extraocular muscles
  - dysthyroid eye disease with diplopia and proptosis (Fig. 19.1);
- Limb muscles
  - up to one-third of patients with hyperthyroidism have evidence of a proximal myopathy,
  - there is also an association between thyrotoxicosis and both myasthenia gravis and periodic paralysis (Chapter 17).

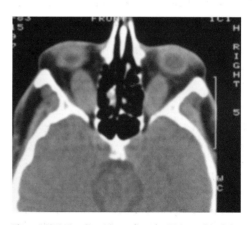

Figure 19.1 Dysthyroid eye disease. CT scan showing gross enlargement of the inferior rectus muscles.

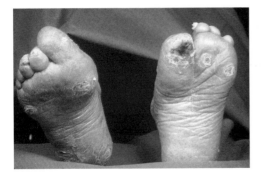

Figure 19.2 Diabetic feet.

Diabetes mellitus

Diabetes mellitus may be complicated by a peripheral neuropathy that can take several forms.

• Distal, predominantly sensory, symmetrical polyneuropathy; the sensory loss may contribute to foot ulcers in diabetic patients (Fig. 19.2) and in extreme instances results in painless arthropathy (Charcot joints, see Fig. 17.5).

• Autonomic neuropathy (Chapter 7).

• Acute painful asymmetrical proximal lower limb wasting and weakness, typically in middle-aged or elderly males, attributed to disease at lumbosacral plexus level (**diabetic amyotrophy** – Fig. 19.3).

• Entrapment neuropathy, e.g. carpal tunnel syndrome (diabetes renders the nerves sensitive to pressure) and other mononeuropathies including cranial nerve palsies (particularly affecting eye movements).

• Various other neuropathies have been described, including a painful neuropathy developing when patients start insulin therapy, thought to be related to axonal regeneration.

The pathogenetic mechanism(s) underlying diabetic neuropathy remain controversial. Disruption of metabolic pathways may exert a toxic influence on nerves, but another important contributing factor is diabetic small vessel disease, including the blood supply of nerves (vasa nervorum), hence the development of mononeuropathies.

Diabetic complications may affect the nervous system by more indirect routes, e.g. vascular disease leading to stroke, and renal failure potentially causing both an encephalopathy and peripheral

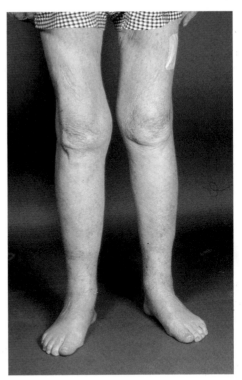

Figure 19.3 Diabetic amyotrophy.

neuropathy. Other causes of acute encephalopathy in diabetes include:

• diabetic ketoacidosis,

• hypoglycaemia – usually related to insulin therapy but sometimes seen with oral hypoglycaemic agents,

• non-ketotic hyperosmolar coma,

• lactic acidosis.

Neurology of pregnancy

Pregnancy may influence the natural history of pre-existing neurological disorders; it may also be associated with specific neurological problems arising anew.

Pre-existing neurological diseases

Epilepsy is often said to follow the 'law of thirds' in pregnancy – one-third deteriorate, one-third improve and one-third are unchanged (in fact, probably a greater proportion are unchanged).

Uncontrolled seizures in pregnancy are potentially damaging to mother and fetus. Anti-epilepsy drugs should therefore be continued throughout pregnancy in patients with recently active epilepsy. Blood levels should be carefully monitored, especially in the third trimester when increased dosage may be necessary. This is particularly the case with lamotrigine, levetiracetam and carbamazepine. For enzyme-inducing drugs, such as carbamazepine, there is an interaction with rising oestrogen levels, which accelerate its metabolism (this interaction is also relevant when carbamazepine is used in patients taking oral contraceptives – higher doses of *both* are generally required). Conversely, in patients where there has been remission of epilepsy for 2 or more years, anti-epilepsy drug withdrawal should be considered before pregnancy is planned. This recommendation relates to the possible teratogenic effects of these drugs. Sodium valproate, in particular, has been associated with an increased risk of neural tube defects (Chapter 18). This risk may be managed by:

- screening in early pregnancy (ultrasound examination, alpha-fetoprotein estimation),
- prophylactic folic acid supplements (5 mg daily) – during pregnancy and indeed now recommended for all women of childbearing age on anti-epilepsy drugs, as the maximum prophylactic benefit is likely to be achieved if folate is being taken at the time of conception.

Vitamin K should be prescribed for the mother in the last month of pregnancy and intramuscularly after delivery to the baby, if the mother is taking enzyme-inducing drugs such as carbamazepine or phenytoin, to prevent haemorrhagic disease of the newborn.

Breast feeding is generally not problematic with the modern anti-epilepsy drugs.

Multiple sclerosis is less likely to relapse during pregnancy, but there is potentially a counterbalancing increased risk of deterioration in the puerperium. Though controversy persists, the overall effect of pregnancy plus the 3-month postpartum period on the natural history of multiple sclerosis is probably neutral. There is, therefore, no basis for the negative recommendations

previously given by neurologists to women with multiple sclerosis contemplating pregnancy. The main factor which should, however, continue to be included in the decision is the capacity of a woman with multiple sclerosis to care for a young child over the years in the face of potentially increasing disability.

Benign tumours, previously clinically silent, may present during pregnancy. These include meningiomas, both intracranial and spinal, which are thought to enlarge because they often express oestrogen receptors. Pituitary adenomas may also swell during pregnancy.

Migraine occasionally poses diagnostic difficulties in pregnancy. Particularly in the third trimester, patients may experience a florid aura, with or without headache. A previous history of migraine and the absence of neurological signs are helpful pointers towards the correct and reassuring interpretation of initially worrying symptoms.

Neurological complications of pregnancy

Pregnancy may trigger disease de novo at several sites in the central and peripheral nervous system.
- Cerebral cortex
  - eclamptic seizures associated with hypertension and proteinuria in pregnancy,
  - stroke, particularly venous sinus and cortical vein thrombosis, for which the puerperium is a risk factor (Chapter 11);
- Basal ganglia
  - dyskinesias may occur with rising oestrogen concentrations (**chorea gravidarum**), hence also seen with oral contraceptives;
- Brainstem and diencephalon
  - Wernicke–Korsakoff syndrome secondary to hyperemesis gravidarum;
- Obstetric neuropathies
  - sciatica as a result of prolapsed lumbar intervertebral disc; similar symptoms may result from pressure on the lumbosacral plexus by the fetal head in the later stages of pregnancy,
  - meralgia paraesthetica (Chapter 17),
  - carpal tunnel syndrome attributed to fluid retention in pregnancy,

- Bell's palsy occurs with increased frequency during pregnancy, particularly the third trimester,
- the location of other neuralgias may suggest involvement of particular nerves, e.g. brachial plexus or intercostal nerves;
- Restless legs syndrome is common in pregnancy.

Neuro-oncology

Malignant disease may affect the nervous system by three major mechanisms:
- direct and metastatic tumour spread to neural and adjacent structures,
- neurological effects of tumours remote from the nervous system (**paraneoplastic syndromes**),
- consequences of treatment.

Tumour invasion and metastasis

Metastatic cancer commonly involves the brain, particularly in the case of primary breast, bronchus and bowel tumours (Fig. 19.4). Intramedullary

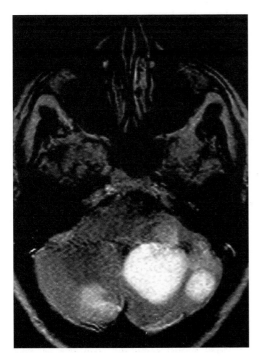

Figure 19.4 MRI showing cerebellar metastases.

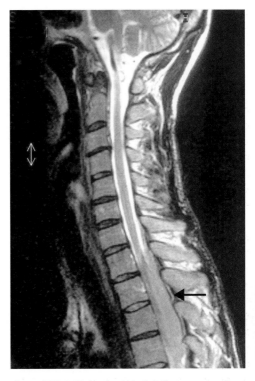

Figure 19.5 MRI showing spinal cord compression due to malignant disease (arrowed).

metastases within the spinal cord are rarer. However, acute cord compression (Chapter 15) may result from vertebral lesions caused by solid cancers which typically spread to bone (breast, bronchus, prostate, kidney, thyroid), and as a result of lymphoma and myeloma (Fig. 19.5). Peripheral nerve infiltration by cancer is rare, but the brachial plexus may be directly invaded by breast or bronchial cancer (Chapter 17). Similarly, the lumbosacral plexus may be infiltrated by pelvic tumours.

Apart from the vertebrae, other structures adjacent to the nervous system that may be invaded by tumours include the spinal epidural space (prostate cancer, lymphoma) and the meninges. **Malignant meningitis** as a result of solid cancers is relatively rare, but lymphoma and leukaemia commonly manifest in this way. Patients present with an 'aseptic meningitis' (Chapter 14) often accompanied by multiple cranial nerve palsies and spinal root lesions. The diagnosis is confirmed by CSF cytology; outlook is poor.

Paraneoplastic disorders

Certain malignancies, particularly carcinomas of the bronchus (small cell type), breast and ovary, and lymphoma, even if not directly spreading to neural structures, may be associated with syndromes at various sites in the nervous system. These uncommon disorders are attributed to the influence of humoral mechanisms, including specific auto-antibodies, provoked by the tumour. Examples include:

• limbic system – inflammatory infiltration may be associated with an amnesic syndrome and seizures ('**limbic encephalitis**'),
• cerebellar ataxia,
• brainstem syndrome with a chaotic eye movement disorder (**opsoclonus**),
• sensory polyneuropathy,
• **Lambert–Eaton myasthenic syndrome** – failure of acetylcholine release at the neuromuscular junction (Chapter 17), associated with small cell carcinoma of the bronchus (a significant minority of patients with this syndrome have no evidence of underlying malignancy but the appearance of the tumour may be delayed, even years after the onset of the neuromuscular disorder),
• dermatomyositis – may be associated with an underlying carcinoma of the bronchus or stomach when presenting in middle-aged men.

Malignant disease may also produce non-metastatic neurological complications by other indirect mechanisms:

• metabolic disorders – hyponatraemia as a result of inappropriate antidiuretic hormone secretion, hypercalcaemia;
• immunosuppression, particularly in leukaemia, lymphoma and their treatment, leading to opportunistic infections, e.g. progressive multifocal leucoencephalopathy (Chapter 14);
• paraprotein production in myeloma associated with a polyneuropathy and also occasionally with hyperviscosity, hence risk of cerebral infarcts. Myeloma neuropathy may also be due to amyloid deposition.

Consequences of cancer treatment

Radiotherapy may be associated with delayed neurological damage (often several years after treatment), particularly radiation plexopathy and myelopathy.

Chemotherapy may produce specific neurological complications, e.g. neuropathy caused by vincristine or cisplatinum.

Connective tissue disorders and other systemic inflammatory diseases

Systemic vasculitis may involve the blood supply of nervous tissue, hence leading to cerebral infarcts, e.g. in systemic lupus erythematosus and polyarteritis nodosa. More commonly, vasculitis affects the vasa nervorum of peripheral nerves, resulting in a multifocal neuropathy ('**mononeuritis multiplex**', Chapter 17), as seen in:

• rheumatoid arthritis,
• systemic lupus erythematosus,
• polyarteritis nodosa,
• Wegener's granulomatosis.

These connective tissue disorders are also associated with other specific neurological complications:

• rheumatoid arthritis – entrapment neuropathies, e.g. carpal tunnel syndrome, cervical myelopathy, especially as a result of atlanto-axial subluxation;
• cerebral lupus – depression, psychosis, seizures, chorea, tremor;
• polyarteritis nodosa – seizures, psychosis, aseptic meningitis, muscle necrosis;
• Wegener's granulomatosis – aseptic meningitis, cranial nerve palsies, intracranial venous sinus thrombosis.

Certain other multisystem inflammatory disorders frequently involve the nervous system:

• Systemic sclerosis – may be associated with polymyositis, and with stroke caused by sclerosis of the carotid or vertebral arteries.
• Sjögren's disease – polyneuropathy, often with cranial nerve involvement, particularly trigeminal sensory loss.

• Sarcoidosis – most commonly presents neurologically with unilateral or bilateral LMN VII nerve palsies. Optic neuropathy may occur, as may peripheral neuropathy and myopathy. Neurosarcoidosis of the CNS, in the absence of systemic disease, may enter the differential diagnosis of multiple sclerosis, as cord lesions occur and the CSF frequently shows inflammatory changes. However, there are some distinctive features of CNS sarcoid, e.g. the tendency for granulomas to involve the hypothalamus, with resultant somnolence and diabetes insipidus.

• Behçet's disease – may present neurologically with a multiple sclerosis-like illness, aseptic meningitis or intracranial venous sinus thrombosis.

The management of all these chronic inflammatory disorders is complex, often involving corticosteroids and immunosuppressant drug regimes. Lesions exerting mass or compressive effect (e.g., large sarcoid granulomas in the cerebral hemispheres, cervical myelopathy in rheumatoid) may be amenable to surgical treatment.

Neurology and psychiatry

The work of neurologists and psychiatrists overlaps in several areas:

• diagnosis and management of 'organic' (see below) psychosyndromes:
  • acute – confusional states (delirium),
  • chronic – dementia;
• management of alcoholism and drug dependence;
• psychological consequences of neurological illness:
  • anxiety and depression secondary to diagnosis of a neurological disorder, e.g. epilepsy, stroke, multiple sclerosis, Guillain–Barré syndrome (Chapter 20), neurodegenerative disease,
  • effects of treatment, e.g. steroid-induced psychosis;
• psychiatric illness manifesting with neurological symptoms.

This last area poses special difficulties of diagnosis and treatment. Some definitions are required:

• **Somatoform disorders** are conditions where physical symptoms, for which no physiological basis exists, are manifestations of underlying psychological conflict.

• **'Functional'** is a term sometimes used to imply symptoms are psychological in origin (i.e. used interchangeably with **psychogenic**). Strictly speaking, however, 'functional' merely means that symptoms are due to changes in organ function rather than structural alterations (in contrast, symptoms relating to changes in structure are termed '**organic**').

Many patients who are anxious experience vague neurological symptoms, e.g. giddiness and paraesthesiae in the extremities, in combination with general medical features such as chest pain, palpitations and dyspnoea, sometimes amounting to a full-blown panic attack. These symptoms are often attributed to unconscious **hyperventilation**. The diagnosis can be confirmed by provoking symptoms by the patient voluntarily overbreathing, and then relieving them by rebreathing from a paper bag.

Hysteria

Vague and non-specific psychogenic symptoms must be distinguished from the phenomenon of hysteria. Here, patients typically exhibit a major loss of neurological function (e.g., paralysis, anaesthesia, blindness, amnesia or apparent loss of consciousness – the last variously termed nonepileptic attacks, pseudo-seizures or hysterical fits) in the absence of an organic cause and in the presence of psychological conflict. Other patients experience multiple symptoms including chronic pain in the absence of physical disease and in the context of personality disorder (polysymptomatic hysteria or **somatization disorder**).

Monosymptomatic hysteria has been analysed on the basis of two psychodynamic mechanisms:

• **Conversion** – where the patient avoids mental conflict by converting anxiety into physical symptoms;

• **Dissociation** – the patient 'splits' the mental self from the physical self.

Either way, the salient feature is that neurological disorder is simulated, but such simulation is thought to be unconscious, as opposed to the conscious mechanisms operating in **malingering** patients. The nomenclature of these conditions is somewhat confused, as the word hysteria has assumed pejorative connotations in many minds. Thus, especially in the psychiatric literature, the terms dissociative or conversion disorders are used interchangeably with hysteria.

Clinical features

Hysteria may be suspected when patients exhibit:
- non-anatomical distribution of weakness or sensory loss, atypical features of a seizure, e.g. unusual sequence of events;
- absence of 'hard' neurological signs, e.g. muscle wasting, reflex changes;
- presence of positive features of simulated dysfunction, e.g. antagonistic contraction in an apparently paralysed limb;
- apparent lack of concern about severe symptoms (**la belle indifférence**);
- evidence of personal gain:
  - **primary gain** – unconscious avoidance of anxiety arising from mental conflict, e.g. as a result of stressful life events,
  - **secondary gain** – care and attention from family, friends and medical and nursing attendants, who may be **manipulated** by the patient.

Management

The diagnosis of hysteria can be difficult. Investigation, if required, should take place immediately after the initial assessment, the patient then being reassured that all the results are normal. Reinvestigation should be avoided.

A non-confrontational approach is probably the most helpful. Initial explanation that stress may cause illness may permit subsequent psychotherapeutic management involving:
- exploration of the underlying psychological conflict,
- behaviour therapy, e.g. reinforcing signs of improvement and ignoring helpless behaviour,
- antidepressants for patients where hysteria is secondary to depression.

In parallel with these measures, a patient with hysterical paralysis should not be refused physiotherapy – it may indeed permit improvement to occur gradually, without the patient 'losing face'.

Chronic fatigue syndrome

Some patients present to neurologists with fatigue as the dominant symptom, present for many months or even years, often together with impairment of concentration and memory. Though fatigue may accompany general medical conditions (e.g., infections, hypothyroidism, malignancy) or neurological disorders (multiple sclerosis, primary muscle disease), these patients have no physical signs of such diseases and the general medical possibilities are eliminated by simple blood tests (full blood count, ESR, thyroid function).

Terminology and aetiology

Patients and the media commonly use the label **myalgic encephalomyelitis** (**ME**) for this syndrome. However, this is a misnomer, as muscle pain, though present in some patients, is by no means universal, and none of these patients has demonstrable inflammation of the brain or spinal cord.

Theories of the cause of the disorder are polarized to two extremes:
- Physical – most patients and their charitable associations, along with some doctors, attribute the syndrome to an organic basis, usually an atypical response to infection (hence yet more confusing nomenclature – **postviral fatigue syndrome**). This notion has arisen in part because some specific viral diseases (notably Epstein–Barr virus) are associated with prominent fatigue in many individuals for months after recovery from the acute infection. However, in many patients with chronic fatigue syndrome, no antecedent viral illness is identified.

• Psychological – many neurologists and psychiatrists have commented on the similarities between the clinical features of chronic fatigue syndrome and those of depression. The condition can therefore be regarded as a type of somatoform disorder, with psychological mechanisms operating as described in the previous section. Patients may be reluctant to accept such interpretations because of the social stigma still attaching to psychiatric diagnoses.

Clinical features

In addition to the major symptoms (fatigue, impaired concentration and memory), patients may present with:
• myalgia – limb or chest muscles,
• joint pain,
• headache, dizziness, paraesthesiae,
• disturbed sleep,
• features of irritable bowel syndrome.

Physical examination is normal. Initial screening blood tests exclude general medical causes of fatigue. Repeated and more extensive investigations are counterproductive.

Management

A non-judgmental, non-confrontational approach is most likely to be helpful. If the patient can be persuaded to take antidepressants (e.g., amitriptyline, dosulepin or newer generation antidepressants such as sertraline in low dosage) and to moderate activity under the guidance of a physiotherapist, with gently graded exercises, improvement is possible even after years of disability.

Key points

• Metabolic encephalopathy presents acutely with a confusional state or coma, sometimes complicated by seizures and movement disorders (tremor, myoclonus, asterixis)
• Thiamine prophylaxis against Wernicke's encephalopathy should be given to at-risk individuals – malnourished alcoholic patients, and those with hyperemesis gravidarum
• Diabetes mellitus may produce many patterns of peripheral neuropathy, e.g. sensory polyneuropathy, autonomic neuropathy, diabetic amyotrophy and pressure palsies
• Pregnancy may alter the course of pre-existing neurological disease, and is also associated with specific neurological complications arising de novo
• Malignant disease may affect the nervous system directly by tumour spread, or indirectly (paraneoplastic disorders)
• Psychiatric disease may manifest with neurological symptoms

---

Multifocal neuropathy in systemic vasculitis

Case history: A 63-year-old woman developed pain in the left leg, rapidly followed by a foot drop and numbness of the dorsum of the foot. Two weeks later, she became aware of pain and tingling in a right median distribution. Within days, her left hand had become weak, with pain and tingling along its ulnar border. In her past history, she had been treated for iritis 2 years previously and had become deaf in the left ear 1 year later. Otoscopic examination at that time had shown a left middle ear effusion. Examination at the time of her neurological presentation revealed normal cranial nerves apart from the hearing loss. In the limbs, there was weakness of the small hand muscles on the left, sparing thumb abduction and opposition. There was also a complete left foot drop, with profound weakness of ankle dorsiflexion and eversion on that side, along with severe weakness of extensor hallucis longus. Her ankle reflexes were absent, plantar responses were downgoing. Sensory testing showed impairment of pinprick and light touch sensation in a right median and left ulnar distribution. Cutaneous sensation was also impaired on the dorsum of the left foot. General examination revealed a 'saddle-nose' deformity. In her initial investigations, there was a normochromic, normocytic anaemia with an ESR of 105 mm/h. Her creatinine was mildly elevated.

Continued on p. 172

Comment: This patient's left peroneal nerve palsy, rapidly followed by right median sensory and left ulnar mixed nerve lesions, indicates a multifocal neuropathy ('mononeuritis multiplex'). The pace of the history, severity, pain and very high ESR strongly suggest ischaemia/infarction of individual peripheral nerves due to vasculitis as the cause. The clues to the specific disease process are the upper airways involvement (saddle-nose deformity, middle ear effusion) and renal impairment, this combination pointing to a diagnosis of Wegener's granulomatosis. Though the diagnosis of this condition can be supported serologically (by the presence of antineutrophil cytoplasmic antibodies), combined nerve and muscle biopsies are warranted (looking for histological evidence of necrotizing vasculitis) before embarking on powerful immunosuppressant treatment with high-dose corticosteroids and cyclophosphamide. Other primary vasculitides associated with multifocal neuropathy include classical polyarteritis nodosa and Churg–Strauss syndrome, the latter comprising the neuropathy, late-onset asthma and eosinophilia.

Hysteria

Case history: A 24-year-old woman woke following a minor gynaecological procedure unable to move her legs, which also felt numb. Continence was preserved. On examination, cranial nerves and upper limbs were normal. In the lower limbs, there was no muscle wasting and tone was normal. Both legs were apparently completely paralysed. Knee and ankle reflexes were normal, and plantar responses were downgoing. On sensory testing, she was unable to detect vibration in the lower limbs and made position sense errors in the feet at a rate greater than would be expected by chance. Cutaneous sensation to light touch and pinprick was reported impaired in both legs with an abrupt circumferential cut-off at the groins. General examination was normal and she seemed remarkably unperturbed by the turn of events. Immediate MR imaging of her brain and whole spine was normal as were nerve conduction studies and EMG. During these studies she was shown that muscles in her legs were able to contract in response to an electrical stimulus. On further questioning, a complex psychosocial background emerged, including a history of sexual abuse in childhood. With a careful, non-confrontational approach, she was able to accept a treatment programme combining graded physiotherapy with psychiatric input and slowly improved.

Comment: The functional basis for this patient's presentation is indicated by the lack of objective abnormal neurological signs, in particular the normal lower limb reflexes. Those signs which were present were subjective, inconsistent and non-anatomical. Additional support for a psychogenic basis is provided by the context, her previous history and her affect of 'belle indifférence'. Important aspects of the management include early thorough investigation which may reassure the patient (and medical staff) and eliminate the need for subsequent reinvestigation, which is best avoided as it would send the patient mixed messages about the medical opinion. A non-confrontational approach is advisable and treatment should combine psychiatric management with physiotherapy, the latter providing the patient with a dignified way out of her predicament. True hysteria is nowadays much rarer than Charcot's and Freud's writings would suggest, but still occurs.

Chapter 20

Neurological emergencies

The management of several acute neurological disorders has been outlined elsewhere in this book in the context of specific disease categories. These include:

- loss of consciousness (Chapter 2),
- raised intracranial pressure (Chapters 9 and 13),
- acute ocular ischaemia, specifically giant cell arteritis (Chapter 9),
- stroke, including subarachnoid haemorrhage (Chapter 11),
- head injury (Chapter 13),
- meningitis (Chapter 14),
- spinal cord and cauda equina compression (Chapter 15),
- metabolic disorders, particularly Wernicke's encephalopathy (Chapter 19).

The remainder of this chapter is restricted to a description of conditions that have not been covered in detail elsewhere and that require specific complex management.

Status epilepticus

Status epilepticus is defined as recurring seizures, without the patient regaining consciousness between attacks, for 30 minutes or more. It is a medical emergency because, if untreated, the

Lecture Notes: Neurology, 9th edition. By Lionel Ginsberg. Published 2010 by Blackwell Publishing.

Table 20.1 Causes of status epilepticus.

Preceding seizure disorder
Non-concordance with medication
Superadded effects of alcohol
No previous seizures
Trauma
Infection (meningitis, encephalitis, abscess)
Tumour
Stroke
Metabolic, hypoxia
Drug overdose, alcohol-related

resultant anoxia may lead to permanent brain damage or death. Management may be divided into three components:

- immediate resuscitative measures – **a**irway, **b**reathing, **c**irculation,
- control of seizures,
- identification (and treatment) of underlying cause (Table 20.1).

Control of seizures is further subdivided according to the clinical stage:

- **Premonitory phase** – diazepam (10–20 mg) may be given intravenously or rectally, repeated once 15 minutes later if status continues to threaten. Alternatively, an intravenous bolus of clonazepam (1–2 mg) may be used.
- **Early status** – the preferred benzodiazepine is intravenous lorazepam (usually a 4-mg bolus) repeated once only, if necessary, after 10 minutes.

- **Established status** – phenobarbitone bolus (10 mg/kg; 100 mg/min) and/or phenytoin infusion (15 mg/kg; 50 mg/min, with ECG monitoring). A benzodiazepine (e.g., clonazepam, 0.5–1.5 mg/h), though carrying a small risk of respiratory depression, may be required to achieve early control while phenytoin is being administered.
- **Refractory status** – if seizures continue for longer than 30 minutes despite the above measures, general anaesthesia should be instituted, using thiopentone (intravenous bolus then infusion). Artificial ventilation is usually required. The anaesthetic dosage should not be tapered until at least 12 hours after the last seizure (which may require EEG monitoring [see below] if the patient is ventilated and hence paralysed with muscle relaxants).

Investigation

Investigation of status epilepticus, as well as being directed towards identification of a cause (Table 20.1), involves:

- EEG
  - to confirm the diagnosis, particularly in refractory cases, which may be functional, i.e. **pseudo-status**, and hence show no EEG abnormality,
  - also (as indicated above), to monitor treatment, titrating anaesthesia until a '**burst-suppression**' pattern is achieved;
- anti-epilepsy drug levels
  - which should be monitored to ensure adequate serum concentrations.

As soon as possible after status has been controlled in a patient with pre-existing epilepsy, their usual oral anti-epilepsy drug regime should be reinstituted (if necessary administered via a nasogastric tube). Maintenance therapy in patients presenting with de novo status depends on the cause.

Acute neuromuscular respiratory failure

Weakness of the ventilatory musculature may occur acutely in diseases of the peripheral nerves or the neuromuscular junction. More rarely, it is due to a central lesion or disorders of the muscles themselves.

By far the most useful lung function test in patients with acute respiratory paralysis is the **vital capacity**. A useful rule-of-thumb cut-off value of 1 L for this variable indicates a need for assisted ventilation. However, patients who are becoming fatigued may best be managed by elective ventilation before vital capacity falls below this arbitrary level.

Guillain–Barré syndrome

Guillain–Barré syndrome is an acute inflammatory demyelinating polyneuropathy (there are axonal variants). In most patients, it is associated with antecedent infection. There is predominant motor involvement, often including the respiratory and bulbar musculature, hence the need for emergency management.

Aetiology and pathogenesis

The cause is incompletely understood, but the pathogenetic mechanism involves inflammatory demyelination with variable axonal damage in the peripheral nervous system. An autoimmune process is presumed to be triggered by various agents (Table 20.2).

Clinical features

Spinal pain and minor sensory symptoms (paraesthesiae in the extremities) may precede progressive, ascending, symmetrical limb weakness. Paralysis of the legs then arms may be followed by cranial nerve involvement with drooling, dysphagia (and nasal regurgitation) and slurred speech. Later still, respiratory muscle weakness,

Table 20.2 Precipitants of Guillain–Barré syndrome.

Viruses	Cytomegalovirus, Epstein–Barr virus, HIV
Bacteria	*Mycoplasma pneumoniae*, *Campylobacter jejuni*
Vaccines	For example, against swine influenza
Surgery	

Table 20.3 Miller Fisher syndrome.

Ophthalmoplegia
Ataxia
Areflexia
Little or no weakness
Association with a specific antiganglioside antibody

Table 20.4 Differential diagnosis of Guillain–Barré syndrome.

Brainstem infarct
Acute spinal cord lesion
Poliomyelitis
Other acute neuropathies, e.g. due to porphyria, vasculitis, drugs, toxins, e.g. lead
Myasthenia gravis
Botulism
Severe myopathy
Hysteria, malingering

with dyspnoea and fatigue, may develop. The course of the illness may be very rapid, with maximum deficit being reached in hours or days – by definition in less than a month. Progression may arrest at any stage, some patients having a relatively mild illness and remaining ambulant, others spending weeks ventilated in an intensive care unit.

On examination, there is flaccid paralysis of the limbs, with early tendon areflexia, and usually only minor sensory deficits. Cranial nerve palsies particularly include the facial nerve and bulbar dysfunction. The **Miller Fisher variant** presents rather differently, with little muscle weakness in the limbs (Table 20.3). Autonomic instability in severe Guillain–Barré syndrome may result in labile blood pressure and cardiac dysrhythmias, along with sphincteric symptoms, e.g. urinary hesitancy and retention and bowel disturbance secondary to ileus.

Investigations and diagnosis

- Lumbar puncture classically reveals a raised CSF protein concentration with normal cell count ('albuminocytological dissociation'), though findings may be normal early in the disease.
- EMG and nerve conduction studies may confirm a demyelinating neuropathy, but again may show only mild or no abnormality at early stages.
- Up to one-quarter of patients will have circulating antibodies to **gangliosides**.

Because these investigations are often negative, other tests may be necessary to eliminate disorders that enter the differential diagnosis (Table 20.4).

Management and prognosis

In the progressive phase of the illness, vital capacity should be measured frequently and the

ECG monitored continuously. Bulbar dysfunction affecting the patient's ability to swallow saliva, or a rapidly deteriorating vital capacity, warrant admission to an intensive care unit, with probable need for artificial ventilation (and nasogastric feeding), if the airway cannot be protected or vital capacity (and oxygen saturation) falls below a critical level. Early tracheostomy aids tracheal toilet and patient comfort.

Limb weakness requires regular physiotherapy, to prevent joint stiffness and contractures, and turning, to protect against pressure sores. Low molecular weight heparin should be administered as prophylaxis against deep vein thrombosis and pulmonary embolism. Mouth and eye care, and aspiration of secretions, need meticulous attention.

Specific immunological treatment is recommended for patients with Guillain–Barré syndrome severe enough to render them non-ambulant:

- plasma exchange, or
- high-dose intravenous immunoglobulins (usually five daily infusions).

These treatments have been shown to speed the rate of recovery and hence reduce the risk of complications. Corticosteroids are ineffective.

Guillain–Barré syndrome is usually a monophasic illness, 80% of patients eventually making a good recovery. However, the time to regaining full independence may be many months, complicated by pain, anxiety and depression, which are under-recognized.

Death occurs in 5–10% of patients, as a result of cardiac dysrhythmia, pulmonary embolism or sepsis consequent on immobility. More than 10% of patients have permanent disability and a few relapse. Indicators of poor prognosis include:

- increasing patient age,
- rapid onset of weakness,
- need for ventilation,
- antiganglioside antibodies,
- preceding diarrhoeal illness,
- electrophysiological parameters showing significant axonal degeneration.

Myasthenic crisis

Myasthenia gravis (Chapter 17) frequently involves the bulbar muscles, and may also affect the diaphragm and intercostal muscles. Acute symptoms in these territories are referred to as a **myasthenic crisis**. This must be distinguished from the situation in myasthenic patients overtreated with anticholinesterases (hypersalivation, lacrimation, increased sweating, vomiting and pupillary constriction in association with muscle weakness and fasciculation – a **cholinergic crisis**).

A myasthenic crisis may occur at any stage in the course of myasthenia gravis in a severely affected patient, but may also be the mode of presentation. The latter situation poses potential diagnostic difficulties – understandable concern about the imme-diate management of a patient's acute respiratory failure often taking precedence over consideration of its cause. The development of acute dyspnoea disproportionate to that anticipated from any co-existent chest infection (which may have precipitated events) in an at-risk individual (e.g., young female), particularly if there is a hint of preceding bulbar symptoms or fatigable weakness elsewhere, should immediately raise suspicion of a myasthenic crisis. Diagnosis may be confirmed by an edrophonium ('Tensilon') test (Chapter 17), where the response may be dramatic, but the test should be conducted with intensive care facilities available. Early management, in addition to protection of the airway and ventilatory support, involves plasma exchange or intravenous immunoglobulin to gain rapid temporary control of the underlying immunological disorder while standard therapies begin to act (Chapter 17).

Key points

- The management of status epilepticus involves the immediate resuscitation of the patient, control of seizures, and the identification and treatment of any underlying cause
- The most useful respiratory function test for monitoring neuromuscular ventilatory failure is the vital capacity; a cut-off value of 1 L indicates a need for assisted ventilation

---

Guillain–Barré syndrome

Case history: A 32-year-old man suffered a diarrhoeal illness. Two weeks after recovering from the gastrointestinal infection, he developed interscapular pain and tingling in his hands and feet. By the next day he was unable to walk, due to leg weakness, and was admitted to hospital. On examination, there was mild bilateral facial weakness, grade 3 weakness in the upper and lower limbs, tendon areflexia, downgoing plantar responses and glove-and-stocking loss of pinprick sensation with impaired vibration sense in the feet. Lumbar puncture showed acellular CSF, protein concentration 1.7 g/L, glucose concentration normal. Initial nerve conduction studies and EMG were normal. The next day he experienced difficulty swallowing and vital capacity fell from 2.7 L in the morning to 1.3 L in the evening. He was transferred to the intensive care unit, electively intubated and ventilated, and treated with high-dose intravenous immunoglobulin.

Comment: This patient shows the typical pattern of severe Guillain–Barré syndrome with antecedent infection (presumably *Campylobacter*), predominant motor involvement despite initial sensory symptoms, 'albuminocytological dissociation' in the CSF and rapid progression to ventilator requirement. Electrical findings are often normal early in the course of the disease but later reveal a typical demyelinating neuropathy. Other important support on the intensive care unit would include ECG monitoring, nasogastric feeding, physiotherapy and nursing care, and measures against venous thromboembolism.

Chapter 21

Neurorehabilitation

Despite advances in drug treatment and surgery, many patients with neurological disorders remain disabled. Disability, which may be static or progressive, has several potential components:

- loss of mobility – as a result of weakness, spasticity, ataxia, extrapyramidal features, sensory loss, dyspraxia;
- incontinence;
- cognitive impairment – dementia, dysphasia, visuoperceptual difficulties;
- psychological factors – anxiety, depression, loss of confidence and motivation;
- chronic pain.

The aim of neurorehabilitation is to restore patients to maximum capability and independence, within the limits set by their disability and their needs. Disability must be distinguished from **handicap**. A mathematician who suffers a spinal injury may be disabled, but not necessarily handicapped in the pursuit of his or her profession.

To achieve the goals of rehabilitation, the development of **multidisciplinary teams**, of which medical and nursing staff form only a part, has proved helpful. Other members of the team, and their roles, include the following.

Lecture Notes: Neurology, 9th edition. By Lionel Ginsberg. Published 2010 by Blackwell Publishing.

Physiotherapy

In the acute phase of major neurological disorders, physiotherapists are primarily concerned with care of the patient's airway and breathing, along with advice about limb positioning. Physiotherapists and nurses are generally better informed than medical staff regarding lifting and moving immobile patients, e.g. transferring from bed to chair. Subsequently, physiotherapeutic input is vital as the patient mobilizes, including management of spasticity, and provision of walking aids (sticks, crutches, frames) and of splints for wrist or foot drop. Gait retraining involves balance exercises for vestibular or cerebellar dysfunction as well as treatment of spasticity and weakness.

Occupational therapy

The assessment of the effects of neurological disability on a patient's everyday activities is the domain of the occupational therapist (OT). A formal checklist is used – the **Activities of Daily Living** – with particular attention to feeding, grooming and bathing, sphincter function and toilet independence, dressing and mobility (including chair–bed transfers, walking or use of wheelchair and ability to manage stairs).

Assessments are initially conducted in hospital departments but home visits are subsequently required. Here the OT may need to advise about structural modifications and aids, e.g. stair lifts, rails. Guidance about types of wheelchair and adjustments to vehicles is also provided by the OT.

Speech therapy

The efficacy of speech therapy in aiding recovery from dysphasia is unproven. However, information and instruction from speech therapists help dysphasic patients and their families to cope with this disability. Speech therapists are also expert in communication aids for patients with severe dysarthria, including provision of electronic equipment that can be used even when there is co-existent limb dysfunction (e.g., in motor neurone disease). A further role for the speech therapist is in the assessment of swallowing. Severe neurogenic dysphagia may warrant bypassing the swallowing mechanism, e.g. by means of a **percutaneous endoscopic gastrostomy**, where a feeding tube is passed directly into the stomach through the abdominal wall.

Neuropsychology

Clinical psychologists are involved in the assessment and diagnosis of patients with cognitive dysfunction (Chapter 3). Some also participate in retraining and counselling brain-damaged individuals.

Social work

Liaison with social services and allied agencies is important before a disabled patient can leave an acute neurological ward. Issues to be decided include whether the patient can return to their former accommodation, with a 'care package' of district nursing services, home helps, structural modifications, etc. Alternatively, rehousing may be required, with varying support, e.g. warden assistance, or a nursing home for severe disability. Social workers also have an important role in financial provisions for disabled patients, advising about appropriate allowances. If patients are not competent to manage their own finances, a suitable individual, e.g. relative, with 'power of attorney' may need to be appointed through established legal channels. A final area of concern is the patient's employment. Neurological disease may leave patients too handicapped to return to their former occupation. Retraining may allow some work to be done. Even if a return to work ultimately seems possible, an extended period of convalescence is usually required after a major neurological illness or injury.

Specific management issues

Paraplegia

Regardless of the cause of a severe spinal cord lesion (e.g., trauma, multiple sclerosis), there are common aspects of the management.

Skin

Pressure sores may develop alarmingly rapidly over bony prominences (e.g., ischial tuberosity, greater trochanter, elbow and heel) in immobile patients, particularly when there is also sensory loss in that area, and when weight loss has occurred. Prevention is vital in at-risk patients – by means of regular careful 2-hourly turning, keeping the skin clean and dry, and use of specially designed mattresses that minimize pressure and friction damage. The management of established pressure sores involves similar principles, along with correction of malnutrition and cleaning the affected area with removal of slough. Sometimes it is necessary to excise the necrotic tissue, with surgical closure or skin grafting.

Bladder

With high spinal cord lesions, patients may develop satisfactory reflex bladder emptying, provided cognitive function and the lower cord and cauda equina are intact, and the bladder wall has not been damaged by recurrent infection and excessive distension. Generally, however, some form of medical intervention is required, depending on the type of bladder disturbance. Two main patterns are recognized, and urodynamic investigations may be needed to distinguish them. The most important investigation is measurement of post-void residual volume.

- **Bladder hyper-reflexia** – with frequency, nocturia, urgency and urge incontinence as a result of loss of inhibition of reflex emptying. If residual volume is <100 mL, treatment consists of anti-cholinergic drugs and antibiotics for any co-existent urinary tract infection.
- **Detrusor–sphincter dyssynergia** – where the hyper-reflexic bladder contracts against a closed sphincter with resultant retention of urine and again risk of infection. Residual volume will generally exceed 100 mL and treatment is by combined use of anticholinergic agents and intermittent self-catheterization.

Early treatment of bladder dysfunction may obviate the need for a long-term indwelling catheter with inevitable intractable urinary infection.

Bowels

Constipation with faecal impaction and overflow incontinence are unfortunately common features of severe spinal cord disease. Early management is essential to avoid these problems. Appropriate measures include:

- adequate bulk in diet – if necessary with supplementary fibre,
- satisfactory fluid intake,
- judicious use of laxatives – many patients are able to establish a regular bowel routine using a combination of an irritant and a lubricant agent,
- avoiding excessive use of opiate analgesics.

Faecal impaction, once present, requires repeated enemas and sometimes manual evacuation of faeces to clear the lower bowel.

Sexual function

Paraplegic patients may not volunteer symptoms of sexual dysfunction and it is advisable to ask specifically about these difficulties, along with providing appropriate information. In this way, unnecessary distress to patients and their partners may be avoided, as many of the problems can be helped.

Erectile impotence has been treated with penile injections of papaverine or prostaglandins, or mechanical vacuum devices, but management has been transformed by oral phosphodiesterase-5 inhibitors, such as sildenafil (see Chapter 16).

In female paraplegic patients, sexual activity may be limited by spasticity, the legs fixed in flexion and adduction. Counselling services and antispasticity measures (see below) may circumvent these problems.

Limbs

Passive movement of paralysed lower limbs is initially important to prevent **contracture** formation. Other simple measures include the use of bed cages to keep heavy bedclothes off the legs and feet, thereby reducing the risk of fixed deformities and superimposed pressure palsies. Prophylaxis against deep vein thrombosis and pulmonary embolism (anti-embolism stockings, subcutaneous heparin) is required in view of the increased risk of these complications consequent on immobility.

Spasticity is best managed in consultation with physiotherapists. The standard drug used in this context is baclofen. It has the disadvantage of reducing spasticity at the expense of increasing weakness but the advantage that it can be administered intrathecally (in specialist units) as well as orally – which may be valuable for treatment of severe lower limb spasticity. Other drugs include dantrolene, diazepam and tizanidine. For very severe spasticity, alternatives to the use of intrathecal baclofen include botulinum toxin injections into affected muscles and, in extreme cases, surgical measures (tenotomy).

Other general medical aspects

Attention to nutrition and fluid intake is important in paraplegic patients, as many of the complications listed previously are exacerbated by weight loss and dehydration. Infection (urinary, chest and from pressure sores) also contributes significantly to morbidity and indeed mortality. The psychological consequences of immobility, particularly depression, are easily overlooked.

Stroke

Many of the considerations relating to paraplegia outlined in the preceding section apply equally to hemiplegia. Patients with major cerebrovascular events are best managed in specialist **stroke units**, where there is an appropriate concentration of multidisciplinary expertise. A similar principle has been applied to the rehabilitation of head injury patients. Stroke units ideally should be equipped to cope with both the acute medical treatment of brain ischaemia and infarction, and longer-term care and rehabilitation. Outside such settings, good management is possible, provided carers are aware of apparently simple principles that are unfortunately easily forgotten in the context of a busy medical ward. Generally, these relate to the correct positioning of the patient. Thus, patients with major non-dominant hemisphere strokes and prominent inattention and neglect may occasionally be found in the corner of a ward with little sensory stimulation, rather than in a position with unrestricted views. Similarly, hemiplegic patients are sometimes seen with the affected arm dangling at their side in internal rotation, with concomitant risk of further morbidity from a frozen or subluxed shoulder, rather than supported on an armrest.

Chronic pain

Chronic pain is defined arbitrarily as pain present continuously or intermittently for 3 months or longer. By this time, treatment may be very difficult; indeed, many patients find their way to a specialist **pain clinic**.

Assuming the patient does not have malignant disease, there are two dominant mechanisms of chronic pain in neurological practice:
- **nocigenic** – as a result of activation of receptors (nociceptors) sensitive to tissue-injuring stimuli,
- **neurogenic** – as a result of dysfunction in the nervous system, in the absence of nociceptor activation.

This distinction is important, as it affects treatment. The differences between nocigenic and neurogenic pain are summarized in Table 21.1. In practice, however, separating pain into these categories may be complicated. For example, nocigenic pain referred from lumbar facet joint dysfunction may mimic the neurogenic pain of sciatica. Furthermore, both types of pain may coexist and both are potentially magnified by psychogenic factors such as anxiety, depression, anger and fatigue.

Drug treatment represents only one aspect of pain relief. Other manoeuvres include:
- physical measures – heat, cold, vibration;

Table 21.1 Nocigenic vs. neurogenic pain.

	Nocigenic	Neurogenic
Examples of causes	Osteoarthritis Lumbar and cervical spondylosis 'Facet joint' pain	Post-herpetic neuralgia Trigeminal neuralgia Central post-stroke 'thalamic' pain Neuropathic, e.g. painful diabetic neuropathy Nerve injury
Clinical features	Sharp, aching or throbbing pain	Burning pain ('ice-burn') Dysaesthesiae Sensory loss Allodynia – pain evoked by stimulus which would not normally be noxious, e.g. light touch
Drug treatment	Analgesics Non-steroidal anti-inflammatory drugs	Tricyclic antidepressants (amitriptyline, dosulepin) Anti-epilepsy drugs (carbamazepine, gabapentin) Topical capsaicin

- acupuncture;
- transcutaneous electrical nerve stimulation (TENS) – particularly for neurogenic pain;
- psychological methods – including relaxation techniques, cognitive behaviour therapy;
- invasive procedures
  - local anaesthetic nerve blocks,
  - sympathetic blockade for partial nerve injuries associated with autonomic dysfunction (Chapter 7),
  - long-lasting nerve lesions (neurolysis) with chemical (phenol, alcohol) or thermal damage, and neurosurgical procedures – usually restricted to pain in advanced cancer.

These various treatments are deployed in a step-wise fashion, using less invasive approaches first. Similarly, drug treatment typically initially involves less potent (and less toxic) agents. Pain clinics provide a setting where patients can receive these pain-relieving measures in a logical sequence and combination, governed by the type and intensity of the pain, and accompanied by appropriate information and advice about the cause of the symptoms. Pain intensity is necessarily subjective, but response to therapy can be monitored reliably using a **visual analogue scale** – the patient at each visit marking a point along an uncalibrated 10-cm line, one end of which represents zero and the other maximal pain.

Key points

- Neurorehabilitation is best achieved by a multidisciplinary team consisting of medical and nursing staff, physiotherapists, OTs, speech and language therapists, neuropsychologists and social workers

---

Multiple choice questions

1. A 23-year-old woman presented with numbness which had ascended from her feet to her waist over the course of 2 weeks. She had also developed urinary urgency and frequency. By the time she was examined, she had started to improve and there were no abnormal signs apart from a sensory level to pinprick at T10.
   What is the most likely diagnosis?
   A. Guillain–Barré syndrome
   B. non-organic symptoms
   C. spinal cord inflammation
   D. spinal tumour
   E. thoracic disc protrusion

2. An 18-year-old man presented with two generalised convulsions, separated by 1 month. He also gave a history that he had been 'clumsy' in the mornings for several years, his arms tending to jerk involuntarily. His uncle had epilepsy. EEG confirmed an epileptic tendency. Brain imaging was normal.
   What is the most appropriate drug treatment?
   A. carbamazepine
   B. ethosuximide
   C. phenobarbitone
   D. phenytoin
   E. sodium valproate

3. A 70-year-old man presented with a 6-month history of visual hallucinations. His sitting room frequently seemed to be full of people. At other times, he was aware that they had not really been there. His wife commented that his memory had also deteriorated, though he still had 'good days'. He was more likely to become confused at night. His mini-mental state examination score was 23/30. On neurological examination, there was poverty of facial expression and mild cogwheel rigidity of the arms, worse on the left.
   What is the most likely diagnosis?
   A. Alzheimer's disease
   B. dementia with Lewy bodies
   C. idiopathic Parkinson's disease
   D. multiple system atrophy
   E. schizophrenia

4. A 63-year-old woman presented with a 3-month progressive history of wasting and weakness of the right hand. On examination, there was wasting, fasciculation and weakness of the interossei and muscles of the thenar eminence on the right. There was a mild increase in tone of the right forearm. The tendon reflexes were brisker in the right arm than the left. Sensory examination was normal.
   What is the most likely diagnosis?
   A. brachial plexopathy
   B. carpal tunnel syndrome
   C. motor neurone disease
   D. T1 motor root lesion
   E. ulnar neuropathy

5. A 47-year-old man presented with an abrupt onset of left-sided headache and double vision. On examination, there was partial left ptosis and impairment of elevation and adduction of the left eye. Depression of the left eye was impaired when it was in the abducted position. The left pupil was larger than the right.

What is the most likely diagnosis?

A. brainstem stroke

B. cluster headache

C. myasthenia gravis

D. ophthalmoplegic migraine

E. posterior communicating artery aneurysm

6. A 67-year-old woman presented with a 2-hour history of left-sided weakness affecting her face, arm and leg. She had previously been well and the weakness had developed suddenly. On examination, she was fully conscious, with mildly slurred speech and profound left-sided weakness. Blood pressure was 130/80 mm Hg. CT head scan was unremarkable with no evidence of haemorrhage.

What is the most appropriate treatment?

A. alteplase

B. aspirin

C. heparin

D. tinzaparin

E. warfarin

7. A 56-year-old man with a history of diabetes mellitus presented with a left foot drop. On examination, there was weakness of left ankle dorsiflexion and eversion, and of dorsiflexion of the big toe. There was also impairment of pinprick sensation over the dorsum of the foot.

Which nerve has been damaged?

A. common peroneal

B. femoral

C. musculocutaneous

D. sciatic

E. tibial

8. A 35-year-old man presented with recurrent severe headaches, each lasting approximately 40 minutes. He had been experiencing 2–3 attacks a day for 1 week, and had been woken by headache in the middle of the night several times. The pain was centred on his left eye and was associated with conjunctival injection, lacrimation and nasal discharge on that side. On examination, there was partial left ptosis and the pupil was smaller on that side.

What is the most likely diagnosis?

A. carotid artery dissection

B. cluster headache

C. medication misuse headache

D. migraine

E. posterior communicating artery aneurysm

9. A 40-year-old woman presented with the visual field defect shown in the diagram below.

What is the most likely site of the lesion?

A. bilateral optic neuropathy

B. above parietal lobe

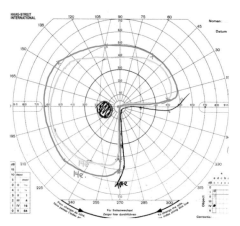

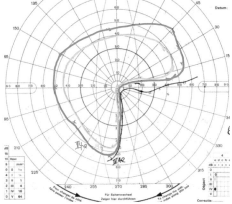

C. above temporal lobe

D. below parietal lobe

E. below temporal lobe

10. A 60-year-old woman presented with an oval patch of numbness and tingling on the lateral aspect of her right thigh. She had recently gained weight. On examination, there were no abnormal signs beyond impairment of pinprick sensation in an area corresponding to the site of her symptoms, above the knee and below the hip.
What is the most likely diagnosis?

A. femoral neuropathy

B. lumbar disc prolapse (L2)

C. meralgia paraesthetica

D. mononeuritis multiplex

E. multiple sclerosis

11. A 68-year-old man in a coma was able to open his eyes to painful stimuli, make incomprehensible sounds and flex (withdraw) his limbs to pain.
What is his Glasgow Coma Scale score?

A. 3

B. 5

C. 8

D. 11

E. 14

12. A 30-year-old man presented with frontal balding, bilateral ptosis and facial weakness. He had difficulty releasing his grip. His father had had cataracts.
What is the most likely diagnosis?

A. Charcot–Marie–Tooth disease (hereditary motor and sensory neuropathy)

B. Duchenne muscular dystrophy

C. dystrophia myotonica

D. mitochondrial myopathy

E. myasthenia gravis

13. A 65-year-old woman was treated for Parkinson's disease with pramipexole.
What is this drug's mechanism of action?

A. dopamine agonist

B. dopamine precursor

C. dopamine release stimulator

D. dopamine reuptake blocker

E. monoamine oxidase B inhibitor

14. A 58-year-old man presented with a 3-month history of asymmetrical pain, wasting and weakness of the thighs. On examination, there was wasting of the right quadriceps more than the left, with weakness of hip flexion and knee extension bilaterally, and absent lower limb tendon reflexes. Vibration sensation was absent at the toes and ankles; pinprick and light touch sensation were impaired in a stocking distribution bilaterally.
Which investigation is most likely to be diagnostic?

A. blood glucose

B. chest X-ray

C. EMG

D. ESR

E. MRI lumbar spine

15. A 27-year-old woman saw zigzag shapes in her left visual field, which spread over the course of 15 minutes, resulting in a complete left homonymous hemianopia which then took a further 15 minutes to resolve.
What is the most likely diagnosis?

A. hypoglycaemia

B. migraine aura

C. occipital epilepsy

D. optic neuritis

E. transient ischaemic attack

16. A 59-year-old man with a history of alcoholism and malnutrition presented in an acute confusional state. He was treated with intravenous fluids and his condition worsened. On examination, he had bilateral sixth nerve palsies, nystagmus and ataxia.
What is the most likely diagnosis?

A. alcohol withdrawal syndrome

B. brainstem encephalitis

C. posterior circulation stroke

D. posterior fossa tumour

E. Wernicke's encephalopathy

17. A 23-year-old woman presented with a
3-week history of progressive difficulty
swallowing and slurred speech. She had
experienced nasal regurgitation of liquids.
Her symptoms were worse in the evenings.
On examination, she had nasal speech,
bilateral ptosis, worse on the left, bilateral
facial weakness, weakness of neck flexion
and of the proximal upper and lower limb
muscles.

What is the most likely diagnosis?

A. dystrophia myotonica

B. Guillain–Barré syndrome

C. motor neurone disease

D. multiple sclerosis

E. myasthenia gravis

18. Which member of the neurological
multidisciplinary team is responsible for a
patient's wheelchair assessment?

A. consultant neurologist

B. occupational therapist

C. physiotherapist

D. social worker

E. ward sister

19. Which member of the neurological
multidisciplinary team is responsible for a
patient's swallowing assessment?

A. occupational therapist

B. physiotherapist

C. social worker

D. speech and language therapist

E. ward sister

20. A 78-year-old woman presented with painful
diabetic neuropathy.

Which would be the drug of first choice to
treat her pain?

A. amitriptyline

B. codeine

C. gabapentin

D. morphine

E. paracetamol

21. Examine this CT head scan (pre- and
post-intravenous contrast, above and below,
respectively).

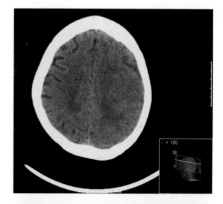

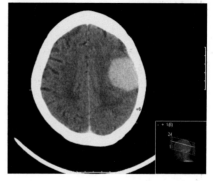

What is the likely diagnosis?

A. cerebral abscess

B. cerebral infarct

C. glioma

D. intracerebral haemorrhage

E. meningioma

22. Examine this CT head scan.

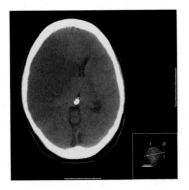

What is the likely diagnosis?

A. cerebral abscess

B. cerebral infarct

C. glioma

D. intracerebral haemorrhage

E. meningioma

23. Examine this CSF profile.

Clear, colourless fluid

Total protein	0.5 g/L (0.15–0.45)
Glucose	4.4 mmol/L (3.3–4.4)
White cell count	180/μL ($\leq$5)
Lymphocyte count	90% (60–70)
Gram stain	No organisms seen

What is the most likely diagnosis?

A. bacterial meningitis

B. Guillain–Barré syndrome

C. subarachnoid haemorrhage

D. tuberculous meningitis

E. viral meningitis

24. Examine this CSF profile.

Clear, colourless fluid

Total protein	2.8 g/L (0.15–0.45)
Glucose	4.4 mmol/L (3.3–4.4)
White cell count	2/μL ($\leq$5)
Lymphocyte count	100% (60–70)
Gram stain	No organisms seen

What is the most likely diagnosis?

A. bacterial meningitis

B. Guillain–Barré syndrome

C. subarachnoid haemorrhage

D. tuberculous meningitis

E. viral meningitis

25. Examine this CSF profile.

Clear, colourless fluid

Total protein	2.8 g/L (0.15–0.45)
Glucose	0.5 mmol/L (3.3–4.4)
White cell count	180/μL ($\leq$5)
Lymphocyte count	90% (60–70)
Gram stain	No organisms seen

What is the most likely diagnosis?

A. bacterial meningitis

B. Guillain–Barré syndrome

C. subarachnoid haemorrhage

D. tuberculous meningitis

E. viral meningitis

Answers to multiple choice questions

1. C – the truncal sensory level and bladder involvement suggest a cord lesion rather than peripheral neuropathy. The improvement is against a structural cause (tumour, disc).

2. E – the combination of generalised convulsions, morning myoclonus and a family history of epilepsy strongly suggests a diagnosis of juvenile myoclonic epilepsy, for which sodium valproate is the treatment of first choice. The situation is more complicated in young women, because of this drug's potential teratogenicity.

3. B – cognitive impairment associated with visual hallucinations, fluctuations with nocturnal confusion, and extrapyramidal signs indicates a diagnosis of dementia with Lewy bodies.

4. C – the weakness extends beyond the distribution of a single peripheral nerve. The presence of upper and lower motor neurone signs in the same limb strongly suggests motor neurone disease, which is often asymmetrical in onset.

5. E – a posterior communicating artery aneurysm compressing the oculomotor nerve may present with a painful 'surgical' third nerve palsy – partial in this case.

6. A – with stroke onset less than 3 hours previously, this normotensive woman with no history of a bleeding tendency is a candidate for thrombolysis with intravenous tissue plasminogen activator (alteplase).

7. A – diabetes renders nerves sensitive to pressure, and this nerve is often compressed as it winds around the fibular neck.

8. B – the periodicity of the attacks and the autonomic accompaniments suggest a diagnosis of cluster headache, which can lead to a full-blown Horner's syndrome, as in this case.

9. B – see caption to Fig. 4.3 for explanation.

10. C – the sensory impairment is in the distribution of the lateral cutaneous nerve of the thigh, which may be compressed as it passes under the inguinal ligament, resulting in the syndrome of meralgia paraesthetica, which is often associated with changes in weight.

11. C – eyes 2, verbal 2, motor 4.

12. C – difficulty releasing grip is a symptom of myotonia. This patient conforms to a classical description of dystrophia myotonica, one of the most common muscular dystrophies to present in adult life.

13. A

14. A – this patient's clinical features are typical of diabetic amyotrophy (diabetic proximal neuropathy). He has a coexistent diabetic distal sensory neuropathy.

15. B – the slow evolution of the visual symptom (minutes rather than seconds or fractions of a second) favours migraine over epilepsy or transient ischaemic attack, as does the description of 'zigzags'.

16. E – the classical triad of ophthalmoplegia, ataxia and confusion, in an at-risk patient, indicates Wernicke's encephalopathy, for which urgent treatment with thiamine, initially intravenously, is required. The patient's condition may have deteriorated in hospital because of intravenous dextrose administration, without concomitant thiamine.

17. E – rapidly progressive bulbar palsy in a young woman, with a history of fatigability, is in keeping with a diagnosis of myasthenia gravis, as is the associated ptosis and facial weakness. Motor neurone disease may also present with progressive bulbar palsy but the patient is in the wrong age group and there are no upper motor neurone signs.

18. B

19. D

20. C – tricyclic antidepressants and anti-epilepsy drugs are more likely to be effective against neurogenic pain than conventional analgesics. In an older patient, gabapentin is likely to be better tolerated than amitriptyline.

21. E

22. B – this scan was performed 4 days after the infarct and considerable swelling is evident, mimicking a tumour, but the density of the lesion is uniformly low and the margins conform to middle cerebral artery territory.

23. E – CSF lymphocytosis with relatively normal protein and glucose.

24. B – raised protein with normal white cell count, the classical 'albuminocytological' dissociation of Guillain–Barré syndrome.

25. D – CSF lymphocytosis with raised protein concentration and very low glucose.

Index

Note: Page numbers in *italics* refer to figures; page numbers in **bold** refer to tables or boxes.